Better Homes and Gardens®

EAT and STAY SLIM

Better Homes and Gardens
EAT AND STAY SLIM

BETTER HOMES AND GARDENS BOOKS
NEW YORK   DES MOINES

CONTENTS

SHOULD YOU REDUCE? 8

Sensible weight control
Signs of overweight

Different body builds
Why reduce?

HOW OVERWEIGHT COMES AND GOES 13

How fat accumulates
Two safe ways to reduce

Automatic calorie counters
Fallacies about reducing

FIGURING YOUR CALORIE NEEDS 16

Daily calorie deficit
Approximate reducing speed

Maintenance calorie chart
Burning calories by exercising

THE ABC's OF SAFE REDUCING 20

Requirements for safe reducing
Elements of good nutrition

Period of greatest weight loss
Losing plateau

FOOD EXCHANGES FOR MENU PLANNING 23

Daily meal plans
Food exchange lists
Packaged exchanges
Serving ideas from each exchange list

Alcohol slows progress
Menu planning steps
Tempting sample menus
85 tested recipes

EATING OUT 74

Tips for private home dinners
Eating in restaurants

Clip-out exchange list
Lunches to carry

FAMILY STYLE REDUCING 81

Family cooking tips
Nutritious meals for everyone

Comparing family and reducer's menu
Snacks and refreshments

HOW TO STAY SLIM 83

Let food exchanges be your guide
Daily exercises
Women: step 1 exercises

Women: step 2 exercises
Men: step 1 exercises
Men: step 2 exercises

INDEX 94

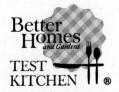

Our checked seal assures you that every recipe in *Eat and Stay Slim* is tested and endorsed by the Better Homes and Gardens Test Kitchen. Each recipe is tested until it measures up to the high standards of family appeal, practicality, and deliciousness.

We are indebted to Donald G. Cooley, noted author on nutrition and medicine, for important contributions made to the development of this book.

FOREWORD

Overweight may be a troublesome problem for the physician to manage, but it can be a devastating situation for the patient. The patient has usually experienced downs and ups in weight. This damages the ego of the physician, and it ruins the self-respect of the patient.

The person properly motivated to lose weight and who understands the probable cause of the overweight has every chance to realize the desired degree of slimness. Frequently, the only ingredient lacking is the means to accomplish that end. Crash diets and grossly imbalanced diets may bring about apparent weight loss, but, all too often weight swoops up again when the dieter goes back to the old patterns of eating. How often can one stand such unsound dieting?

Now, at last, there's a sound approach to weight control, an approach which stresses the importance of variety and balance—the keys to good nutrition. EAT AND STAY SLIM emphasizes that calories do count but it does the counting for you. The dieter simply chooses food items and, like a computer, the plan tabulates the calories and balances the diet. The time and medically proven food exchange system is here expertly explained in what must be the clearest presentation to date. Dietitians and doctors are trained to use the food exchange system for the calculation and planning of the diabetic diet. The patient discussing the plan with the doctor will therefore find a friendly ally in the book. The doctor and the book speak the same language.

The reader may find the food exchange system somewhat challenging at first glance but illustrations, color coding, and cross reference will quickly clear up any problems. Once mastered, use of the exchange system in menu planning will become second nature. When this happens, the dieter can get off the dieting roller coaster for good.

Planned, regular exercise is also a necessary ingredient in a weight control program. Exhilarating physical activity uses up calories, improves the tone of sagging muscles and helps to develop vital respiratory and circulatory reserves. Exercise, to be effective, must be quite vigorous. For many people, a program of exercises takes the place of vigorous sports activities. When time and space are problems, a program of exercise like those developed by the President's Council on Physical Fitness, serves quite well. EAT AND STAY SLIM includes highlights of the Council's program.

EAT AND STAY SLIM provides the educational goal so often absent from books and plans for weight control—a sensible plan for weight maintenance. The information in this book will be useful to all who are interested in nutrition and health.

Readership should not be restricted to those with weight problems. This is a book for all people.

Philip L. White, Sc.D.
Secretary
Council of Foods and Nutrition
American Medical Association

CHAPTER 1

SHOULD YOU REDUCE?

Eat and stay slim—whether you're already slim (and trying to stay there) or just contemplating becoming more sylphlike. The formula is simple: eat tasty, nutritious meals and enjoy every minute of it. There's no catch. Many delightful years of eating and staying slim lie ahead.

First of all, ask your doctor if you should reduce (if he hasn't told you already). If he says to reduce, you should. No ifs or buts about it.

Why go to a doctor at all about such an obvious problem as overweight? Why not just plunge into the latest fad reducing diet and get it over with without bothering your doctor? There are several reasons why not.

Fad diet lore

Perhaps the most important reason is that some faddist or makeshift diets extol one to two foods, allegedly bursting with slimming "miracles," or stress one class of foods at the expense of others. This can result in omission or insufficiency of other classes of foods which provide essential nutrients.

Diets excessively "high" in one thing or in another—high-fat, high-protein, high-carbohydrate—can as well be looked on as "low" in something else. Restrict your carbohydrate intake excessively and you'll likely be on a high-fat diet without knowing it.

Weight control is not a matter of crash reducing for brief periods of time. It's a lifetime matter and the foods you reduce on should be the kind you'd love to live with forever.

Another reason for consulting a doctor is that his physical checkup will determine what ails you, if anything, besides overweight. He may discover some condition that requires treatment, independently of overweight.

Believe it or not, a few people who are already beanpole slim want to reduce because emaciated models with sunken eyes look soulful and glamorous to them. A doctor can prevent such dangerous folly by giving sound medical advice, if he's listened to.

Telltale bulges

To reduce safely you must have excess fat to lose. Generally, excess fat is all too visible to the eye. And the public eye. But you can "measure" it privately. Stand with nothing on in front of a full-length mirror. Look for telltale bulges, such as fleshy pads or "spare tires." Fat tends to cluster in slightly different areas in men and women:

Women: under chin, back of neck, breast, abdomen, upper arm, buttocks and hips, thighs.

Men: under chin, back of neck, abdomen, trunk.

Stand erect, sink your chin into your chest, and look downward. If you can't see your toes without craning your neck you have something to lose.

Tense your abdominal muscles as if someone were aiming a blow at you.

While doing this, press your fingertips over your midriff. If the fat pad over underlying muscles feels soft and cushiony, you could spare some of it. A physically fit person should be able to feel the hardness of tensed muscles and even see a nice muscular ripple or two.

The "pinch test" gives another clue to excess fat. Lie flat, relax, dig thumb and finger into a fatty area, and pinch. This gives a gauge to the thickness of fat over muscle.

Do last year's clothes have shrinking fits? Have your waistline and neckline measurements increased in the last 5 years or so? If you're more than 25 years old, could you get into the clothes you wore then? Has the width of your shoe size increased? Do buttons and zippers have that strained look?

Such signs may persuade you that you have fat to spare. Another way is

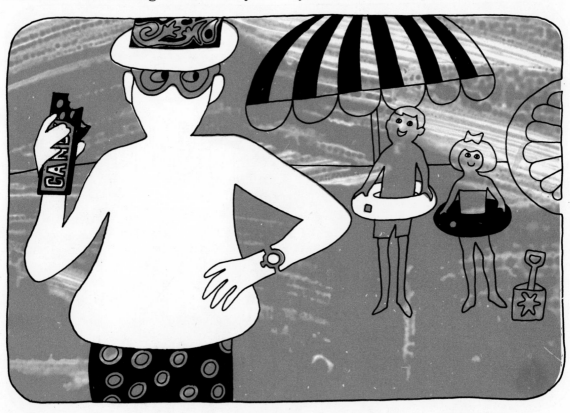

to check your standing in a weight chart. Standards of desirable weight, based on findings of a government study, are on page 11 for women and on page 12 for men.

Big bones and muscles can affect proportions of fat to total weight. You've doubtless recognized different body builds all your life, without giving them a name. "Small," "medium," and "large" frames are the titles used by the government study. In this way they allow for individuality in weight of bones and muscles. It's safer to underestimate than to overestimate the heft of your frame. Chances are that if your actual weight exceeds your desirable weight by 10 pounds or more, your doctor will tell you it's time to reduce.

Rarely, excess weight may not be excess fat. Large amounts of water (which weighs more than fat) may ac-

cumulate in the tissues and tip the scales. Abnormal water retention is usually associated with some physical disorder. Just another reason to consult your doctor before you start a reducing program of any kind.

Why reduce?

Better personal appearance is a wonderful reason for keeping your weight normal, but there are other reasons. Obesity is frequently associated with onset of diabetes in susceptible persons, and with high blood pressure. Excess fat makes breathing less efficient and puts a cruel load on joints that have to support it. Besides, overweight people usually have a shorter life span. General fitness—get-up-and-go—is usually improved when useless dead weight is taken off vital organs.

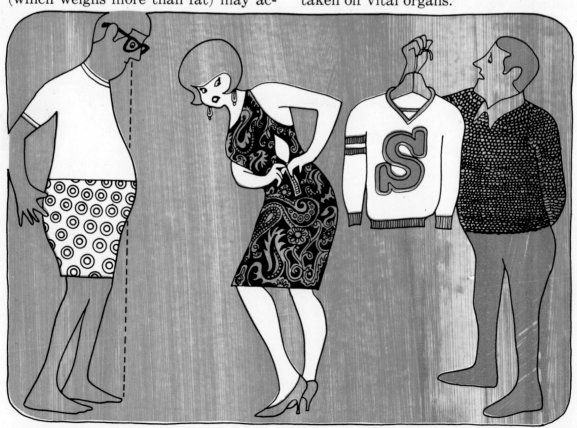

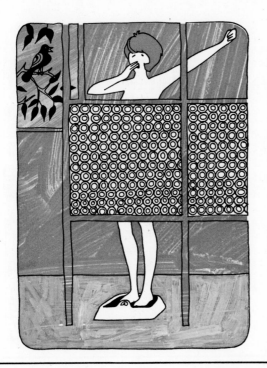

The chart below adjusts the recommended weight according to different body builds. The body build refers to the size and weight of the bone structure in comparison to the height. A woman with larger bones and muscles should naturally weigh more than a woman with smaller, more delicate bones. Persons with small frames are shorter than the average and have small shoulders, hips, anklebones, and wrists. The person with a large frame has wide shoulders, thick wrists, and is taller than the average. Most people have average or medium frames.

The measurements in this chart are without shoes and clothing. Your weight should fall close to the desirable weight for your height.

WOMEN
DESIRABLE WEIGHTS FOR HEIGHT

HEIGHT	SMALL FRAME	MEDIUM FRAME	LARGE FRAME
60 *inches*	100 *pounds*	109 *pounds*	118 *pounds*
61 *inches*	104 *pounds*	112 *pounds*	121 *pounds*
62 *inches*	107 *pounds*	115 *pounds*	125 *pounds*
63 *inches*	110 *pounds*	118 *pounds*	128 *pounds*
64 *inches*	113 *pounds*	122 *pounds*	132 *pounds*
65 *inches*	116 *pounds*	125 *pounds*	135 *pounds*
66 *inches*	120 *pounds*	129 *pounds*	139 *pounds*
67 *inches*	123 *pounds*	132 *pounds*	142 *pounds*
68 *inches*	126 *pounds*	136 *pounds*	146 *pounds*
69 *inches*	130 *pounds*	140 *pounds*	151 *pounds*
70 *inches*	133 *pounds*	144 *pounds*	156 *pounds*
71 *inches*	137 *pounds*	148 *pounds*	161 *pounds*
72 *inches*	141 *pounds*	152 *pounds*	166 *pounds*

In the chart below the desirable weight for men is adjusted according to different body builds and height. Judge the body build by the height of a man and the size of the wrists, anklebones, hips, and shoulders. If a man is tall and has large shoulders and wrists, he has a large frame. Naturally he should weigh more than a short man with smaller wrists, anklebones, and hips. Most men have average or medium frames.

The measurements in this chart are without shoes and clothing. Your weight should fall close to the desirable weight for your height. If you have any question concerning your weight, check with your doctor. In men, excess weight tends to accumulate under the chin, back of neck, abdomen, and trunk.

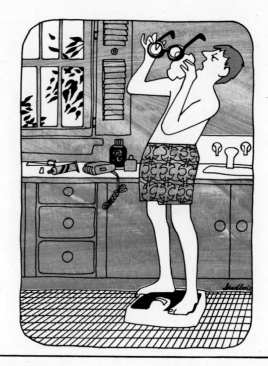

MEN
DESIRABLE WEIGHTS FOR HEIGHT

HEIGHT	SMALL FRAME	MEDIUM FRAME	LARGE FRAME
63 inches	118 pounds	129 pounds	141 pounds
64 inches	122 pounds	133 pounds	145 pounds
65 inches	126 pounds	137 pounds	149 pounds
66 inches	130 pounds	142 pounds	155 pounds
67 inches	134 pounds	147 pounds	161 pounds
68 inches	139 pounds	151 pounds	166 pounds
69 inches	143 pounds	155 pounds	170 pounds
70 inches	147 pounds	159 pounds	174 pounds
71 inches	150 pounds	163 pounds	178 pounds
72 inches	154 pounds	167 pounds	183 pounds
73 inches	158 pounds	171 pounds	188 pounds
74 inches	162 pounds	175 pounds	192 pounds
75 inches	165 pounds	178 pounds	195 pounds

CHAPTER 2

HOW OVERWEIGHT COMES AND GOES

How does excess body fat pile up where it's not wanted?

It comes from eating more food than we burn up by physical activity and bodily processes that require energy to run on.

Here's the how of it: foods furnish heat energy that is measured in units called calories. If we take in more calories from food and drink than we burn up by activity and basic body functions, the surplus calories are stashed away in the form of body fat. They have no other place to go. It's a sort of fat-bank. If excessive intake of calories continues, the fat-bank bulges and bulges from an excess of deposits. And it shows.

Reducing is a matter of making *withdrawals* from the fat-bank. Like an ordinary savings account, the fat-bank shrinks and disappears if we take out more than we put in.

There are only two safe and natural ways to do this: (1) eat less, to reduce calorie intake; or (2) increase physical activity, to burn up more calories.

Either way, calorie *deficit* can be produced. Extra calories the body needs are withdrawn from the fat-bank, which then shrinks.

Theoretically, an overweight person could eat as usual and reduce by running around the block a certain number of times every day. Increased exercise is an important aid to reducing, not to say general fitness. But it's not very practical or easy as a sole means of shedding fat. Successful reducing almost always requires reasonable restriction of food intake. In short, it requires a low-calorie diet combined when possible with a little more activity to help you slim faster and feel better at the same time.

That's what this book is all about.

Automatic calorie counters

Your body never fails to count a calorie, whether you do or not. It's not necessary to look up calorie tables when you plan meals. It's much easier to let Food Exchanges count calories

14

for you—a very pleasant relief indeed.

As explained on page 23, Food Exchanges are units, long used by professional dietitians, of the variety of foods —meats, vegetables, fats, fruits, etc.— that are foundations of good nutrition. The Food Exchanges furnish definite amounts of calories. So, in planning meals, Food Exchanges not only help to balance the diet, and allow personal choices of foods you like, but also count your calories automatically.

One thing about it, you're *sure* to shed excess fat if your calorie deficit is sufficient to make withdrawals from your fat-bank. If this weren't true, we'd get fatter and fatter while starving to death on nothing but air and water. It's well to remember that everything that makes fat enters via the mouth. That's where fat control begins. And all too often ends.

Fallacies about reducing

Misconceptions about reducing explain the appeal of many get-slim-quick schemes which seem to promise that the self can be made into a sylph by magic with no effort at all.

Novel diets of supposedly superior slimming-power keep springing up and fading away. Sometimes it is implied that the calories of certain foods or beverages are totally ignored by the body. But calories always count, whatever their source. The only ones that don't are those you don't swallow. Sometimes, incredible virtues are attributed to exotic foods, or to one or two foods at the expense of others, although common wholesome foods in variety are the best and safest foundations for reducing diets.

Massage, by hand or with vibrators,

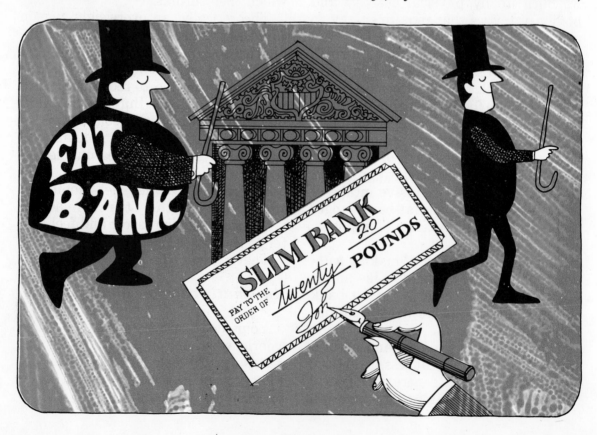

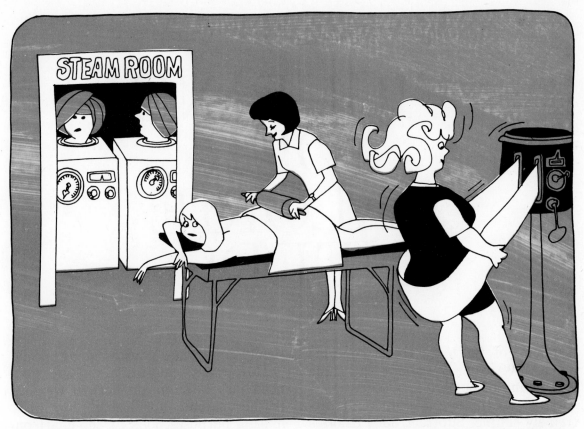

has valuable uses, but not for reducing. Fat won't rub off. Local deposits can't be reduced by rollers or by shaking, shimmying gadgets. If so-called "spot reducing" measures seem to get results, it's because the subject has been made to eat less, or get more active exercise, or both. Passive exercise (the kind in which all the effort is provided by another person, or by a motor-driven machine) is useless for shedding fat or increasing muscle strength. It may make you feel good, though.

Water is part of total body weight. Sweating, from exercise, a hot bath, or baking in a steam cabinet, can get rid of a pound or two of weight in a hurry. But it's merely water which is promptly replaced when you take a drink. Body fat can't be steamed off.

"Reducing pills" prescribed by doctors are potent drugs, available on prescription only. Most common pills act on centers of the brain to depress appetite. This may make a low-calorie diet more satisfying during the first few weeks when the reducer is adjusting to it and learning better eating habits.

Another drug prescribed by physicians is thyroid substance, which makes body fires burn more brightly. Persons who produce too little thyroid hormone of their own may be sluggish and overweight, and thyroid supplements can make up the deficiency. However, if a person's thyroid production is normal (tests are necessary to determine this) additional thyroid substance can be hazardous. Most overweight people have normal thyroid function.

The place of drugs in weight reduction is very simple. If your doctor prescribes them, take them. If he doesn't, just leave them alone.

CHAPTER 3

FIGURING YOUR CALORIE NEEDS

A pound of fat body tissue contains about 3500 calories—about the same as a pound of butter.

So the arithmetic of reducing is extremely simple. Subtract 3500 calories and you shed a pound of fat. Subtract 7000 and you shed 2 pounds.

Of course this takes a bit of doing. But it's heartening to know that it needn't, or shouldn't, be done all at once. You can set your own reducing speed, within limits.

Take in 1000 fewer calories a day than you burn up and you should lose about 2 pounds in a week—about the maximum rate of fat loss that most doctors think desirable without close medical supervision. Or you can subtract only 500 calories a day, and lose about a pound a week.

Actual weight loss on a reducing diet may be greater or less than you expect and may have its ups and downs. There are modifying factors such as water retention (see page 22). But the difference between caloric intake (food) and output (energy expenditure) basically determines your reducing speed.

How many calories a day do you need just to maintain normal weight, neither gaining nor losing? For estimating purposes, look at the chart on the opposite page.

Overweight people use a few more calories to maintain their overweight. There are individual differences of size and shape, and variations of the caloric needs of the same person, but for practical purposes the figures give a yardstick of desirable caloric intake by men and woman who aren't doing pole vaults or playing basketball all day long. These are *maintenance* calories. To shed fat, you'll have to cut down on your caloric intake.

For instance, if you're a normally active woman, 25 years of age, weighing 121 pounds, figure it like this:

Maintenance calories	2000
Subtract calories furnished by a reducing diet	1500
Daily calorie deficit	500

The body burns 2000 calories, gets 1500 of them from the diet, and the remaining 500 from fat stores of the body. That's what makes the fat go away. To get the approximate reducing speed, divide the daily calorie deficit into 3500 calories per pound of fat body tissue. This equals the number of days it takes to lose a pound of fat body tissue. For the woman in our example it would be figured as follows:

$$3500 \div 500 = 7 \text{ days}$$

Weight loss usually is greater because some water is lost with the fat.

Choose one of the food exchange reducing plans of 1000, 1200, or 1500 calories (page 27) and estimate your reducing speed as explained above. You can't be exact to the last ounce or even half pound, but you can come close enough. Ultimately, your body is the most infallible calorie-counter of all and will tell you positively how you're doing.

More exercise, less fat

Would you like to lose fat just as fast on a 1500 calorie diet as on a 1000 calorie diet?

It could be done by increasing your physical activity 500 calories' worth. Like walking at a fast clip for an hour and a half.

That may be more exercise than you care for. An easier route to slimness is reduction of food intake. But you may not be able to win a lifetime victory over overweight unless you combine an increase of physical activity with reduction of caloric intake.

One reason fat tends to accumulate

MAINTENANCE CALORIE CHART

Desirable Weight **Daily Maintenance Calorie Allowance**

MEN	25 YEARS	45 YEARS	65 YEARS
121 lbs.	2450	2200	1850
132 lbs.	2600	2350	1950
143 lbs.	2750	2500	2100
154 lbs.	2900	2600	2200
165 lbs.	3050	2750	2300
176 lbs.	3200	2900	2450
187 lbs.	3350	3050	2550
198 lbs.	3500	3150	2600

WOMEN	25 YEARS	45 YEARS	65 YEARS
99 lbs.	1750	1600	1300
110 lbs.	1900	1700	1450
121 lbs.	2000	1800	1550
128 lbs.	2100	1900	1600
132 lbs.	2150	1950	1650
143 lbs.	2300	2050	1750
154 lbs.	2400	2200	1850
165 lbs.	2550	2300	1950

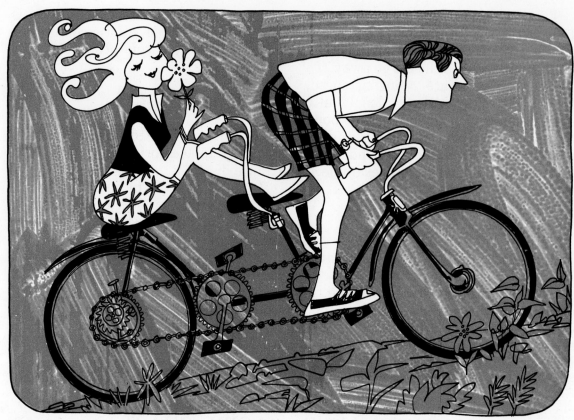

after age 25 is that body metabolism and physical activity tend to dwindle but food intake stays the same. Thus pounds can pile up slowly without increased food intake. Along with a reduction of caloric intake, increased activity helps to restore balance in favor of the slim figure.

It is surprising how many calories can be burned off by a relatively small daily increase of exercise. A brisk walk around the block for 20 minutes burns only 100 calories. But keep it up every day for five weeks and you subtract the equivalent of one pound of fat body tissue—or 3500 calories.

Exercise "mystery" solved

Differences in physical activity explain some of the supposed "mysteries" of overweight. For instance, an obese woman may say: "I eat less than my slim friends but still gain weight. It must be my glands." It is quite possible that she does gain weight while eating less than others who do not gain. But glands rarely have much to do with it.

One study of overly fat women showed that they actually ate *less* than comparable women of normal weight. But they also spent about two-thirds less time in activities involving significant amounts of exercise. Another study of overweight adolescent girls showed that they spent much less energy during "exercise" periods than their slim counterparts. In fact, they coasted a lot.

Overweight women in these studies didn't exercise off as many calories as normal-weight women. Consequently, they got fat although they weren't enormous eaters. They simply took in more calories than they burned. There was no great "mystery" about it.

Burning calories by exercising

Here are estimates of the calories burned per hour by a 154 pound man doing several kinds of activities:

activity	calories/hour
Bicycle riding, moder- ate speed	175
Dancing, foxtrot	266
Horseback riding, trot	301
Skating	245
Swimming, 2 miles/hr.	553
Table tennis	308

However, the calorie-cost of exercise varies with intensity of performance. Very few people swim for an hour at top speed. Some people burn more calories while sitting than others. The lean ones fuss and twitch, change position, gnash their teeth, grip a pencil tightly. More placid, and more upholstered, people just sit and relax.

To figure how a little added exercise can help you stay slim, let's take a fairly measurable form of exercise—walking at 3.5 miles an hour— and see how much this gets rid of in terms of familiar foods:

Food	Extra calories burned by walking at 3.5 m.p.h. for:
Large apple	20 minutes
2 slices bacon	18 minutes
Glass of beer	22 minutes
Doughnut	30 minutes
Boiled Egg	15 minutes
Hamburger	70 minutes
Apple pie (1/6)	75 minutes
Ice cream soda	50 minutes
Soft drink	20 minutes

What kind of exercise?

Regular exercise is far better than occasional bursts of strenuous activity. Things we enjoy doing are best because things we like are habit-forming and exercise should become a habit that we don't have to nudge ourselves into grudgingly because it's "good for us." Walking, swimming, lawn-mowing, dancing, spading the garden—you name it and it's fine as long as you stop short of fatigue.

Formal sitting-up exercises done in a routine way have their place, too. They won't remove fat from certain spots and those spots alone. To the extent that calisthenics increase your expenditure of calories, they cause a general rather than a local loss of body fat. For pleasant daily exercises to help you stay slim see page 85.

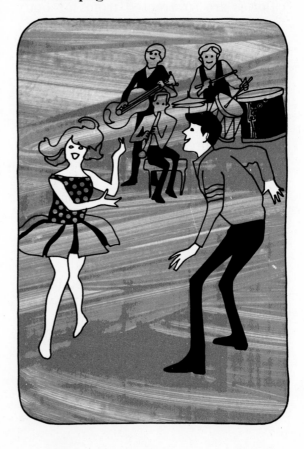

CHAPTER 4

THE ABC's OF SAFE REDUCING

A low-calorie diet usually does not provide as many calories as the body burns in its activities. To make up this deficit, calories are subtracted from fat body tissue. Thus the first requirement for safe reducing is that you have excess fat body tissue to lose. Otherwise, a low-calorie diet could "steal" from vital organs, muscles, tissues—in other words, the real "you."

As we have seen in discussing calorie needs, the presence of excess fat body tissue is usually all too apparent to yourself and to others. If there is the slightest doubt, ask your doctor.

The second requirement is that your diet provide all essential nutrients *except* calories. Minerals, protein, vitamins and other elements must be replenished daily. A well-balanced reducing diet of wholesome foods provides ample amounts of these nutrients.

The trick is to provide the nutrients while at the same time cutting down on calories. This is not very difficult, and certainly is not mysterious. When using food exchanges you can devise scores of slimming menus using familiar foods from your own kitchen and refrigerator. These diets are custom-made to your own taste and convenience. They are just as effective as and safer than some diets which list specific foods—for example a lamb chop or dish of apricots for lunch or dinner. You may not have lamb chops or apricots around. In fact you may not even like these foods. With food exchanges it doesn't matter. You can instantly substitute an equivalent Meat and Fruit Exchange from what you have on hand or like better. At the same time it automatically gives the framework for well-balanced diets of desired caloric value.

Elements of good nutrition

Protein is of primary importance to all living things. It is essential for growth and repair of tissues, for providing the spark that speeds chemical activities of body cells. The foods which furnish top-quality protein are of animal origin. In the food exchange sys-

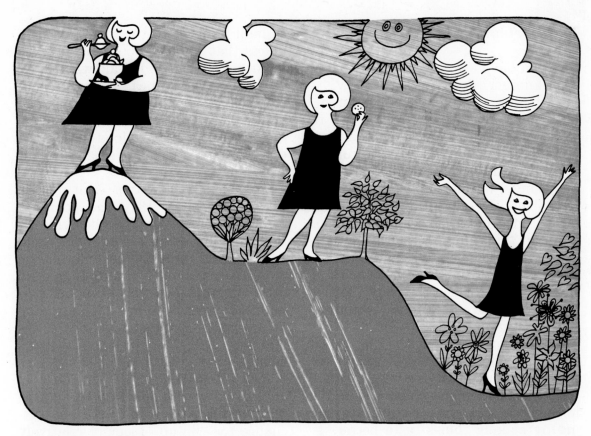

tem, these foods are found in the Meat and Milk Exchanges.

Fats and oils (liquid fats) are essential in the diet. They provide "staying power" to meals, and weight for weight contain more than twice as many calories as carbohydrates or proteins. This can make them deceptive; they can load a menu with more calories than reducers expect. Much of the fat we eat is "invisible," in meats, dairy products, and eggs, or is added in the preparation of foods.

Carbohydrate foods (starches, sugars) furnish most of the energy for moving and living. They free protein for other uses, make use of fat more efficient, and are inexpensive, important carriers of vitamins and minerals. Most of our carbohydrates come from vegetables, cereals, and fruits. Dairy products furnish some, meats virtually none.

What to expect when reducing

Diets can be standardized but people can't. Individual factors such as amount of exercise or water retention can affect the apparent speed of reducing. It is quite possible to lose *fat* although for a time the scales may show little or no *weight* loss.

Allowing for individual variation, experienced physicians generally agree on some broad truisms about reducing:

• The greatest weight loss for most people on a reducing diet usually occurs during the first week, major weight loss during the first month.

• Weight loss may hit a plateau and level off at the end of 4 to 6 weeks. Don't be discouraged. It's probably a good sign that the body is adapting to a lower calorie intake, which is needed to maintain your weight loss.

Fluid retention

If you have less weight loss one day than another, don't be surprised. Expect it. Few reducers show consistent, unvarying weight loss from week to week. The scales may show considerable fluctuation, up today, down tomorrow. Often this is a fluid matter, reflecting changes in salt and water balances of the body. Every pint of retained fluid equals one pound of weight (not fat). This can "hide" fat loss that has actually occurred. Generally, fluid fluctuations are greatest in the first stages of reducing, after which the body "settles down" and the scales more truthfully reflect actual fat loss.

Restriction of salt in the diet tends to give a more even rate of weight reduction. Common salt is a weighty matter. It holds a certain amount of water in the body and tends to stimulate eating by making things taste better. It also provokes thirst and fluid intake. Retained fluids may be not only plain water, but soft drinks and other beverages containing calories (watered-down calories may be deceiving, but count the same as "solid" ones).

Altogether, it's a good idea to go easy on the saltcellar and to avoid highly salted foods such as potato chips and popcorn when reducing.

For that satisfied feeling

A well-balanced reducing diet is never a "starvation" diet for anyone with fat to lose. The so-called "hunger pangs" of reducing are usually due not to hunger, but to appetite, quite a different matter. Here are several ways to stretch a low-calorie diet into a lot of eating satisfaction:

Fragment your meals. You don't have to limit yourself to three meals a day, unless that satisfies you. You can distribute your daily food allowance into 4, 5, or 6 small meals to keep your stomach satisfyingly busy. In that way you make good use of nature's original appetite depressant, food. A snack doesn't count extra if it's part of your daily diet quota.

Take your time. Savor each morsel, take small bites. Play the gourmet, connoisseur of flavors. This delaying action can slow down eating momentum which could propel you into eating more than you really want. It takes a little time for food you have eaten to inform you that you are filled up. Stop before you're satiated and wait a few minutes for the message "that's enough" to come through.

Bulky foods help to prolong the meal and give time for filled-up feelings to register. See As Desired Vegetable Exchange for "fill-up" foods of relatively few calories.

Don't eat when you're not hungry. Silly advice? Well, have you ever eaten bridge-game tidbits for the same reason that men climb mountains, "because they're there"? Or taken a piece of cake to please a hostess? Or nibbled to pass the time away?

Artificial sweetners can be useful adjuncts to a reducing diet when used as directed. All they contribute is sweet flavor, but this can be consoling when concentrated sugars are limited in your diet and carbohydrate comes mainly from cereals, fruits, and vegetables.

Weigh first thing in the morning, after urination and before eating and drinking. It's the most encouraging time, since you've slept off an ounce or so during the night. For added incentive, score your progress by filling out the weekly weight record on page 96.

CHAPTER 5

FOOD EXCHANGES FOR EASY MENU PLANNING

Don't let the term *Food Exchange* intimidate you. It looks pretty technical. In fact, for many years it has been a technical aid for dietitians who must carefully balance diets for patients.

But there's nothing formidable about the food exchanges in this book. All the analysis has been done for you, to make it simple to reduce and stay reduced while doing away with the fuss and bother of calorie-counting, balancing calculations, and all that.

Each food exchange is merely a measurement of calorie and nutrient values. One *Meat* Exchange, for example ¼ cup tuna, furnishes the same amount of protein, fat, and calories as 5 oysters. Thus the two can be interchanged on a menu without changing the calorie count. That, basically, is why they are called food "exchanges." A Meat Exchange isn't necessarily meat. It can be peanut butter or cheese or an egg all delivering about the same amount of nutrients and calories.

Foods are not exactly alike, but they fall into 8 groups, each of which has similar amounts of protein, fat, carbohydrate, and calories. These groups are Meat, Bread, As Desired Vegetables, Sturdy Vegetables, Fruit, Milk, Fat, and a group of "free" foods good for tickling your palate or filling you up without adding significant calories. You can choose any food within a group when planning menus. That is why the 8 groups are called FOOD EXCHANGE LISTS—any food within each list can be exchanged for another. Any difference of calories of foods within a group is adjusted by the *amount* of a food serving.

Thus, the food exchange plan simplifies reducing by:
• Counting calories for you.
• Assuring a well-balanced diet by including different food groups that have different virtues.
• Permitting you to choose, within a food group, the foods you like best or have on hand—you never have to run out for something special.
• Providing menus easily adapted for family members.

Using the food exchange lists

Look at the Food Exchange Lists (pages 28-31). Included foods are every-day bulwarks of the American diet. Each list has a color symbol for quick-as-a-glance recognition. The whole square represents 1 Food Exchange.

- 1 Meat Exchange
- 1 Bread Exchange
- As Desired Vegetable Exchange
- 1 Sturdy Vegetable Exchange
- 1 Fruit Exchange
- 1 Milk Exchange
- 1 Fat Exchange
- Free Exchange

The size of each serving is specified. Meat Exchange units are given by weight, all others by standard measuring cup and spoons.

At first glance, some foods in an exchange list may seem out of place. Why is an egg a Meat Exchange? Because it delivers about the same cargo of protein, fat, and calories as meat. You'll find sherbet, "starchy" vegetables, and even ice cream (for which you deduct 2 Fat Exchanges from the full day's menus) listed as Bread Exchanges. Do we mean that you can substitute sherbet for a cereal if you feel like it? Absolutely! That's pretty handy, especially if you have sherbet on hand but no cereal. Or vice versa. What could be more flexible? Bread Exchanges are quite high in carbohydrate and deliver a modest amount of protein. Again, the exchange unit is a uniform package of calories and nutrients.

Vegetable Exchanges are divided into As Desired and Sturdy groups. The As Desired ones have a high water content, negligible calories, and you can eat them to your heart's, or stomach's, content. Sturdy vegetables, as the name suggests, are a little higher in carbohydrate, protein, and calories.

Milk Exchanges include only fluid milk and dried milk solids (cheese is a Meat Exchange). Fat Exchanges, besides familiar fats and oils, include nuts, olives, avocados, cream, and salad dressings because they're pretty fat.

Not at all hard to understand, is it? Now you're ready to put the food exchange reducing plan to work.

Easy meal planning

The Daily Meal Plans (page 27) give you a choice of three "reducing speeds" —1000, 1200, or 1500 calories a day. Choose a meal plan giving a daily calorie deficit that lets you reduce no more than two pounds a week (see page 16-17). From now on, think no more about counting calories.

Just select the foods you like from the respective food exchange lists specified for each meal. For example, on a 1000 calorie diet you are allowed 1 Fruit Exchange for breakfast. The Fruit Exchange List (printed in part, below) gives many choices—½ small banana, 2 large fresh figs if you feel exotic, or ½ cup applesauce if you don't.

FRUIT EXCHANGE

Raw, cooked, canned unsweetened, or frozen unsweetened
- Apple, 1 (2-inch diameter)
- Applesauce, ½ cup
- Apricots, dried, 4 halves
- Apricots, fresh, 2 medium
- Banana, ½ small
- Blackberries, 1 cup
- Blueberries, ⅔ cup
- Cantaloupe, ¼ (6-inch diameter)
- Cherries, sour, ½ cup
- Cherries, sweet, 10 large
- Dates, 2
- Figs, dried, 2
- Figs, fresh, 2 large

Go down all the other specified food exchanges for breakfast, lunch, and dinner and make your choices. One Meat Exchange is equivalent to 1 ounce of meat. You are allowed 3 Meat Exchanges for lunch and 3 at dinner.

■	1 Meat Exchange	= 1 ounce trout
+ ■	1 Meat Exchange	= 1 ounce trout
■	1 Meat Exchange	= 1 ounce trout
■ ■ ■	3 Meat Exchanges	= 3 ounces trout

So you can have 3 ounces of trout or chicken or ham, or you can split the 3 Meat Exchanges (printed in part, below) as suits your fancy—maybe an egg and a slice each of bologna and cheese.

MEAT EXCHANGE

- ■ Cheese
  American, Cheddar, Swiss: 1 ounce slice, 1 inch cube, ¼ cup grated
  Cottage, not creamed, ¼ cup
- ■ Cold cuts, 1 slice
  4½-inch diameter, ⅛ inch thick
  Bologna
  Braunschweiger
  Luncheon loaf
  Minced ham
  Salami, Cotto
- ■ Eggs, 1
- ■ Fish
  Cod, halibut, haddock, trout, snapper, etc., 1 ounce cooked
  Crabmeat, lobster, ¼ cup
  Sardines, 3 medium
  Shrimp, clams, oysters, 5 small

You may be allowed only ½ of a Milk Exchange. If so, choose any item from the Milk Exchange List but cut the quantity in half.

■	1 Milk Exchange	= 1 cup skim milk
◣	½ Milk Exchange	= ½ cup skim milk

For ½ Milk Exchange you may have ½ cup of skim milk, for instance, instead of the 1 cup for a full exchange.

MILK EXCHANGE

- ■ Buttermilk, from skim milk, 1 cup
- ■ Dried skim milk powder, ¼ cup
- ■ Dried whole milk powder‡, ¼ cup
- ■ Evaporated milk‡, ½ cup
- ■ Evaporated *skim* milk, ½ cup
- ■ Homogenized or whole milk‡, 1 cup
- ■ Plain yogurt‡, 1 cup
- ■ Skim milk, 1 cup
- ■ 2% butterfat milk**, 1 cup

‡Omit 2 Fat Exchanges from diet.
**Omit 1 Fat Exchange from diet.

Your selections will automatically add up, in round numbers, to the number of calories in the meal plan you choose. The number of food exchanges specified in your Daily Meal Plan takes care of that. What a relief to make gourmet choices of your favorite foods instead of counting calories!

Remember, you can substitute one food for another in the *same* food exchange list, which has the same color symbol. But you can't substitute foods of one exchange list for foods of a different exchange list, without risk of upsetting dietary balance or calorie contribution. You can't exchange grapefruit juice for cottage cheese. Foods of a color flock together—with the same color symbol, that is.

The Daily Meal Plans show the conventional 3 meals a day. But there's no law about it. You can divide your allowed food exchanges for the day into half a dozen small meals, or 3 meals and a coffee break or bedtime snack. If you carry a lunch you might want to use a dinnertime bread allowance in order to have a lunchbox sandwich.

"Mixed" foods, such as stews, combine foods from different exchange lists. Their composition can be calculated closely enough by "dissecting" them into the Milk, Vegetable, Meat, or other Exchanges that go into them. This procedure was used to calculate the different exchanges in packaged foods (see Packaged Exchanges, page 31). For recipes see pages 52-73. This dissecting doesn't always give you enough calories or nutrients to equal 1 Food Exchange. As a result ½ Food Exchanges and ¼ Food Exchanges are used. Look for the following symbols:

■ 1 Milk Exchange
◣ ½ Milk Exchange
▲ ¼ Milk Exchange

For example on page 70, one serving of Frozen Orange Dessert equals ¼ Milk Exchange. You have 1 Milk Exchange for lunch on all 3 "reducing speeds." By drinking ¾ cup skim milk and eating 1 serving of Frozen Orange Dessert you have 1 Milk Exchange.

Built-in daily variety

Endless variety is built into the Daily Meal Plans. Take full advantage of it in making your food exchange choices. Variety comes pretty near to being a magic word in nutrition. Too much of one type of food, too little of another, makes a diet lopsided.

The Daily Meal Plans furnish a fine balance of essential nutrients in the most convenient way. You can substitute foods that you happen to have on hand, that are in season and inexpensive when plentiful, or that you just happen to like best. If there's no bread in the house, but there is a small boiled potato in the refrigerator, it's nice to know that you can substitute the potato for bread. Making such choices from the food exchange lists makes for variety in a mixed diet. The Daily Meal Plans are good mixers.

To hold your weight loss

The Daily Meal Plans are deficient only in calories (that's why they make excess fat disappear). After you have reduced to your ideal weight, you will need more calories—well, probably not a great deal more—to maintain it without putting a load of fat back on your frame again.

With your eating habits geared to weight reduction, it should be easy to increase your caloric intake to maintenance levels (see "How to Stay Slim," page 83). You can use the Daily Meal Plans as the foundation of a balanced diet. For example, while keeping the same balance of good nutrition, you can increase the calories by adding a few extra servings from the different food exchanges. You will recognize the values of the different food exchanges almost instinctively by the time you reach the happy stage when you need more calories to keep from wasting away to a shadow.

Don't forget, exercise is just as important to a maintenance diet as it is to a reducing diet. So, keep in shape.

REMEMBER THESE POINTS.

One Food Exchange: A measurement of calorie and nutrient values. Foods within the same exchange list can be interchanged.

Food Exchange Lists: Eight lists of foods having similar amounts of protein, fat, carbohydrate, and calories. The different caloric value of foods is adjusted by the *amount* of a food serving (pages 28-31).

Daily Meal Plans: A daily guide of reducing plans which counts calories for you (page 27).

Daily meal plans

FOOD EXCHANGES AND COLOR SYMBOLS	1000 calories a day number of exchanges	1200 calories a day number of exchanges	1500 calories a day number of exchanges
BREAKFAST			
Meat Exchange	1	1	1
Bread Exchange	1	1	1
As Desired Vegetable	any amount	any amount	any amount
Fruit Exchange	1	1	1
Milk Exchange	½	½	½
Fat Exchange	1	1	2
Free Exchange	as desired	as desired	as desired
LUNCH			
Meat Exchange	3	3	3
Bread Exchange	—	1	2
As Desired Vegetable	any amount	any amount	any amount
Fruit Exchange	1	1	1
Milk Exchange	1	1	1
Fat Exchange	—	1	2
Free Exchange	as desired	as desired	as desired
DINNER			
Meat Exchange	3	3	3
Bread Exchange	—	1	2
As Desired Vegetable	any amount	any amount	any amount
Sturdy Vegetable	1	1	1
Fruit Exchange	1	1	1
Milk Exchange	½	½	½
Fat Exchange	—	1	2
Free Exchange	as desired	as desired	as desired

Choose a meal plan giving a daily calorie deficit that lets you reduce no more than two pounds a week (see pages 16-17). And think no more about calories.

Just select the foods you like from the respective food exchange lists (pages 28-31) specified for each meal. Your daily menu will have endless variety.

Food exchange lists

The Food Exchange Lists are eight groups of foods containing similar amounts of protein, fat, carbohydrate, and calories. The foods included are everyday favorites of the American diet. Each list has a color symbol for quick-as-a-glance recognition. The specified serving amount listed for each food item is equal to one food exchange.

Using a Daily Meal Plan on page 27, select foods you like from the respective Food Exchange Lists specified for each meal.

Your selections will automatically add up, in round numbers, to the number of calories in the meal plan you choose. Remember, you can substitute one food for another in the *same* food exchange list.

■ MEAT EXCHANGE ■

■ Cheese
    American, Cheddar, Swiss: 1 ounce, 1
        slice, 1 inch cube, ¼ cup grated
    Cottage, not creamed, ¼ cup
■ Cold cuts, 1 slice
    4½-inch diameter, ⅛-inch thick
    Bologna
    Braunschweiger
    Luncheon loaf
    Minced ham
    Salami, Cotto
■ Eggs, 1
■ Fish
    Cod, halibut, haddock, trout, snapper,
        etc., 1 ounce cooked
    Crabmeat, lobster, ¼ cup
    Sardines, 3 medium
    Shrimp, clams, oysters, 5 small
    Tuna, salmon, ¼ cup
■ Frankfurter, 1
■ Peanut butter, 2 tablespoons

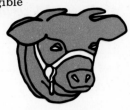

1 MEAT EXCHANGE EQUALS
Carbohydrate, negligible
Protein, 7 grams
Fat, 5 grams
Calories, 73

■ Meat, poultry (no bone or visible fat)
    1 ounce cooked or 3¼x2x¼-inch slice
    Beef
    Chicken
    Corned beef
    Ham
    Lamb
    Liver
    Pork
    Turkey
    Veal

■ FREE EXCHANGE ■

May be used in any amount desired.
■ Bouillon
■ Broth, clear, fat free
■ Coffee
■ Cranberries
■ Gelatin, low-calorie
■ Gelatin, unflavored
■ Lemon
■ Mustard
■ Non-caloric sweetener,
    liquid, powder, or tablets
■ Pepper
■ Pickles, dill, unsweetened
■ Pickles, sour
■ Rennet tablets

1 FREE EXCHANGE EQUALS
Carbohydrate, negligible
Protein, negligible
Fat, negligible
Calories, negligible

■ Rhubarb
■ Spices
■ Tea
■ Vinegar

■ FRUIT EXCHANGE ■

Raw, cooked, canned unsweetened, or
frozen unsweetened

- Apple, 1 (2-inch diameter)
- Applesauce, ½ cup
- Apricots*, dried, 4 halves
- Apricots*, fresh, 2 medium
- Banana, ½ small
- Blackberries, 1 cup
- Blueberries, ⅔ cup
- Cantaloupe†*, ¼ (6-inch diameter)
- Cherries, sour, ½ cup
- Cherries, sweet, 10 large
- Dates, 2
- Figs, dried, 2
- Figs, fresh, 2 large
- Grape juice, ¼ cup
- Grapefruit†, ½ small
- Grapefruit juice†, ½ cup
- Grapes, 12
- Honeydew melon, ⅛ (7-inch diameter)
- Mango†*, ½ small
- Nectarine, 1 medium
- Orange†, 1 small
- Orange juice†, ½ cup
- Papaya†, ⅓ medium

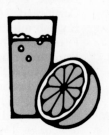

1 FRUIT EXCHANGE EQUALS
Carbohydrate, 10 grams
Protein, negligible
Fat, negligible
Calories, 40

- Peach, 1 medium
- Pear, 1 small
- Pineapple, ½ cup cubed or 1 slice
- Pineapple juice, ⅛ cup
- Plums, 2 medium
- Prunes, dried, 2 medium
- Raisins, 2 tablespoons
- Raspberries, 1 cup
- Strawberries†, 1 cup
- Tangerine, 1 large
- Watermelon, 1 cup

†Rich sources of vitamin C.
*Rich sources of vitamin A.

■ FAT EXCHANGE ■

- Avocado, ⅛ (4-inch diameter)
- Bacon, crisp, 1 slice
- Butter or margarine, 1 teaspoon
- Diet-type margarine, 2 teaspoons
  (For table use only, don't use in cooking.)
- Cream, whipping (40%), 1 tablespoon
- Cream, light (20%), 2 tablespoons
- Cream cheese, 1 tablespoon
- French or Italian salad dressing,
  1 tablespoon
- Mayonnaise, 1 teaspoon
- Nuts, 6 small
- Oils or shortening, 1 teaspoon

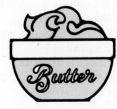

1 FAT EXCHANGE EQUALS
Carbohydrate, negligible
Protein, negligible
Fat, 5 grams
Calories, 45

- Olives, green, 5 small
- Sour cream, 1 tablespoon

■ MILK EXCHANGE ■

- Buttermilk, from skim milk, 1 cup
- Dried skim milk powder, ¼ cup
- Dried whole milk powder‡, ¼ cup
- Evaporated milk‡, ½ cup
- Evaporated *skim* milk, ½ cup
- Homogenized or whole milk‡, 1 cup
- Plain yogurt‡, 1 cup
- Skim milk, 1 cup
- 2% butterfat milk**, 1 cup

‡Omit 2 Fat Exchanges from diet.
**Omit 1 Fat Exchange from diet.

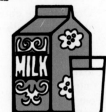

1 MILK EXCHANGE EQUALS
Carbohydrate, 12 grams
Protein, 8 grams
Fat, negligible
Calories, 80

■ BREAD EXCHANGE ■

- Bread, white, rye, whole wheat, 1 slice
    Biscuit, 1 (2-inch diameter)
    Cornbread, 1½-inch cube
    English muffin, ½
    Frankfurter bun, ½
    Hamburger bun, ½
    Melba toast, 7 rounds or 4 slices
    Muffin, 1 (2-inch diameter)
    Roll, 1 (2-inch diameter)
- Cake, plain and unfrosted angel
    or sponge, 1½-inch cube
- Cereal
    Cooked, ½ cup
    Dry, flaked or puffed, ¾ cup
- Crackers
    Graham, 2 (2½-inch square)
    Oysterettes, 20 (½ cup)
    Round, thin, 6 to 8 (1½-inch diameter)
    Rusks, 2
    Saltines, 5 (2-inch square)
    Soda, 3 (2½-inch square)
- Flour, 2½ tablespoons
- Ice Cream, ½ cup
    (omit 2 Fat Exchanges)
- Noodles, spaghetti, cooked, ½ cup
- Rice or grits, cooked, ½ cup

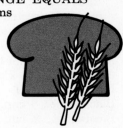

1 BREAD EXCHANGE EQUALS
Carbohydrate, 15 grams
Protein, 2 grams
Fat, negligible
Calories, 68

- Sherbet, ⅓ cup
- Vegetables
    Baked beans, no pork, ¼ cup
    Beans and peas, dried, cooked, ½ cup
        black-eyed peas, kidney, lima, navy,
        split peas
    Corn, popped (plain), 1 cup
    Corn, sweet, ⅓ cup or ½ ear
    Lima beans, fresh, cooked, ½ cup
    Mixed vegetables, ½ cup
    Parsnips, ⅔ cup
    Potato, white, 1 (2-inch diameter)
        baked or boiled
    Potato, white, mashed, ½ cup
    Sweet potato or yam, ¼ cup

■ AS DESIRED VEGETABLE EXCHANGE ■
Any amount may be eaten at each meal.

- Asparagus
- Bean sprouts
- Beans, green or wax
- Broccoli*†
- Brussels sprouts
- Cabbage
- Cauliflower
- Celery
- Chickory*
- Cucumber
- Eggplant
- Endive
- Escarole*
- Greens, all kinds*
    beet, chard, collard, kale, mustard, spinach
- Lettuce
- Mushrooms
- Okra
- Parsley
- Pepper, green*†
- Pimiento
- Radish
- Romaine
- Sauerkraut

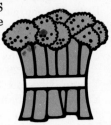

1 AS DESIRED VEGETABLE EXCHANGE EQUALS
Carbohydrate, negligible
Protein, negligible
Fat, negligible
Calories, negligible

- Squash, summer
- Tomatoes*
- Vegetable juice cocktail

■ STURDY VEGETABLE EXCHANGE ■
One serving equals ½ cup cooked
vegetable or ½ cup raw vegetable.

- Artichoke
- Beets
- Carrots*
- Onions
- Peas, green
- Pumpkin*
- Rutabaga
- Squash, winter*
    Butternut, acorn
- Turnip

*Rich sources of Vitamin A.
†Rich sources of Vitamin C.

1 STURDY VEGETABLE EXCHANGE EQUALS
Carbohydrate, 7 grams
Protein, 2 grams
Fat, negligible
Calories, 36

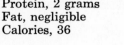

Packaged exchanges

CRACKERS

Multi-shaped crackers, 11, ■ 1 Bread Exchange and ▨ 1 Fat Exchange

Onion-flavored crackers, 10, ■ 1 Bread Exchange and ▨ 1 Fat Exchange

Round cheese crackers, 6, ■ 1 Bread Exchange and ▨ 1 Fat Exchange

Shredded wheat wafers, 3, ■ 1 Bread Exchange

Small pencil-shaped Cheddar cheese crackers, 8, ◣ ½ Bread Exchange

Thin pretzel sticks, 30, ◣ ½ Bread Exchange

Thin triangle shaped crackers, 14, ■ 1 Bread Exchange and ▨ 1 Fat Exchange

3-ring pretzels, 6, ■ 1 Bread Exchange

Wheat wafers, 7, ■ 1 Bread Exchange

For plain crackers see Bread Exchange List.

MISCELLANEOUS

Carbonated beverages, low-calorie, less than 5 calories per bottle, ▨ Free Exchange

Cranberry-juice cocktail, low-calorie, ½ cup, ▨ Free Exchange

Cranberry sauce, low-calorie, ½ cup, ■ Free Exchange

Croutons, 1 cup, ■ 1 Bread Exchange

Dessert topping mix, low-calorie, prepared according to package directions, ⅓ cup, ▨ 1 Fat Exchange

Fish sticks, frozen, 3 sticks, ■ 1 Bread Exchange and ■ ■ 2 Meat Exchanges

Gelatin dessert, low-calorie, plain, ▨ Free Exchange

Mayonnaise, low-calorie, 2 tablespoons, ▨ 1 Fat Exchange

Pudding, low-calorie, made with skim milk according to package directions, ⅔ cup, ■ 1 Milk Exchange

Salad dressings, less than 5 calories per tablespoon, commercial bottled, French, Italian, etc., ▨ Free Exchange

Soy sauce, ▨ Free Exchange

Tomato paste, 3 tablespoons, ■ 1 Sturdy Vegetable Exchange

Tomato sauce, ¼ cup, ■ 1 Sturdy Vegetable Exchange and ▨ 1 Fat Exchange

Vegetables, frozen in butter or cream sauce, ½ cup, ■ or ▨ Appropriate Vegetable Exchange and ▨ 1 Fat Exchange

SOUP

The following soups may be used in unlimited amounts as they are a ▨ Free Exchange:

Bouillon   Consomme   Clear broth

Other soups may be used in exchange for foods allowed in your diet. The following list shows the Exchanges for ½ *can of condensed soup* (before milk or water is added to the soup). Use milk in soups from the Milk Exchange.

Beef, ■ 1 Bread Exchange and ■ 1 Meat Exchange

Beef noodle, ■ 1 Bread Exchange

Black bean, ■ ■ 2 Bread Exchanges

Chicken gumbo, ■ 1 Bread Exchange

Chicken noodle, ■ 1 Bread Exchange

Chicken rice, ■ 1 Bread Exchange

Chicken vegetable, ■ 1 Bread Exchange and ▨ 1 Fat Exchange

Clam chowder, Manhattan-style, ■ 1 Bread Exchange and ▨ 1 Fat Exchange

Cream of asparagus, ■ 1 Bread Exchange

Cream of celery, ■ 1 Bread Exchange and ▨ 1 Fat Exchange

Cream of chicken, ■ 1 Bread Exchange and ▨ 1 Fat Exchange

Cream of mushroom, ■ 1 Bread Exchange and ▨ ▨ 2 Fat Exchanges

Cream of potato, ■ 1 Bread Exchange

Green pea, ■ ■ ◣ 2½ Bread Exchanges

Minestrone, ■ 1 Bread Exchange and ▨ 1 Fat Exchange

Onion soup, ■ 1 Bread Exchange

Pepper pot, ■ 1 Bread Exchange and ■ 1 Meat Exchange

Scotch broth, ■ 1 Bread Exchange and ▨ 1 Fat Exchange

Tomato, ■ 1 Bread Exchange and ▨ 1 Fat Exchange

Turkey noodle, ■ 1 Bread Exchange

Vegetable, ■ 1 Bread Exchange

Vegetable beef, ■ 1 Sturdy Vegetable Exchange and ■ 1 Meat Exchange

Vegetarian vegetable, ■ 1 Bread Exchange

Contributions to this list were made by the Greater Boston Diabetes Society, Inc.

Meat exchange

Meat Exchanges are protein keystones of your meals. They make sure that you get enough tissue-building, tissue-repairing protein of high quality. Meat Exchanges provide generous amounts of B vitamins, minerals such as iron and phosphorus, some fat, but very little carbohydrate.

In most meals, the meat course is the piece de resistance, generally the most expensive item, and other food exchanges must be added to furnish what Meat Exchanges don't. But Meat Exchanges aren't all meat, poultry, or fish. Eggs, cheese, peanut butter, allow a wide variety of personal choices of top-notch protein foods. And they all taste good.

Serving ideas

• Any shortening or butter used to brown ■ meat must be counted as a ■ Fat Exchange. Pans with non-stick surfaces eliminate the need for fat in browning.
• Flour for dredging meat or thickening gravy is from the ■ Bread Exchange. ■ Meats brown satisfactorily without a flour coating. Try serving the ■ skimmed pan juices instead of thickened gravy.

• To add new zest to ■ meats, use the Main Dish Seasoning Guide on page 58. Add ■ seasonings in small amounts. Start with ¼ teaspoon for each four servings; then taste before adding more. Try a combination of seasonings. Good seasoning will enhance the natural flavor of food, not disguise it.
• Brush ■ meat with ■ commercial bottled low-calorie dressing before broiling, or add ■ Worcestershire sauce or ■ soy sauce to cooking liquid.
• Serve ■ cheese shredded atop ■ pear salad, sliced for a ■ cheese and ■ fruit dessert tray, or cubed for snacks.
• ■ Cottage cheese accompanies ■ fruit, or is stuffed into ■ tomato cups. To dress up salads or cooked vegetables, try adding hard-cooked ■ eggs, sliced or halved.
• For breakfast try an ■ egg cooked in a non-stick pan or soft boiled or poached. Or substitute ■ peanut butter on your ■ toast. Another time, broil a slice of ■ ham or ■ Canadian bacon.
• Use ■ Meat Exchanges as an appetizer: ■ Shrimp with ■ Seafood Cocktail Sauce (page 53) or ■ cheese-stuffed ■ celery are tasty ways to start a meal.

For a late evening snack serve a giant wedge of ■ Cheddar or star-studded ■ Edam with an assortment of ■ crackers. Join in the fun by saving ■ 1 Meat Exchange and ■ 1 Bread Exchange from meal plan. Then you can eat 1 ounce of cheese and 5 saltines.

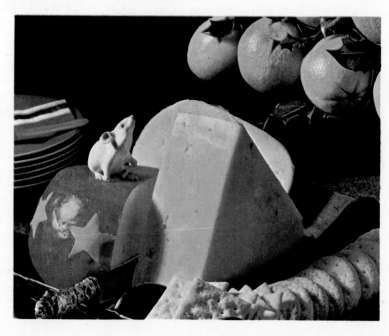

Bread exchange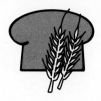

Here are your daily packets of energy. Bread Exchanges, together with vegetables and fruits, furnish carbohydrate (sugars and starches) which is the primary fuel for moving muscles and keeping body fires burning. If we don't get enough carbohydrate, the body has to make it as needed from proteins or fats. Carbohydrate saves protein for better and more important uses. It also helps us to burn fats more efficiently.

Breads and cereals (especially the enriched kinds) give us important B vitamins and minerals necessary for body functions. Potatoes have a little vitamin C, and sweet potatoes a good deal of vitamin A.

There is almost no fat in Bread Exchanges, which is good news for calorie-savers. The protein content of Bread Exchanges (except dried peas and beans) is not high, nor is it as good a source as the protein of Meat and Milk Exchanges, but it is nevertheless important and constitutes a major source of protein for many peoples of the world.

Concentrated sugars and syrups are almost pure carbohydrate, and less desirable for reducers than cereals, fruits, and vegetables which furnish other vital nutrients as well.

Serving ideas

• Serve an assortment of ▪ crackers as an accompaniment with soups and salads or with ▪ cheese or ▪ peanut butter for a snack. ▪ Graham crackers plain or spread with ▪ peanut butter make a good bedtime snack with a glass of ▪ milk.
• Combine ▪ cereals with ▪ milk and ▪ fruit for a tasty breakfast treat. ▪ Non-caloric sweetener will add a sweet touch.
• Some of the more "starchy" vegetables are also part of the ▪ Bread Exchange. ▪ Corn is great roasted over the coals to a caramel color or Mexican style from the can. ▪ Dried peas or beans go into the hearty, long-cooking winter soups.
• Dessert treats include ▪ sherbet, ▪ ice cream (omit ▪ ▪ 2 Fat Exchanges from diet), ▪ sponge cake, and ▪ angel cake. By eating sherbet instead of ice cream you can save ▪ ▪ 2 Fat Exchanges for other uses. Lemon, lime, pineapple, or raspberry sherbet is tasty combined with fresh or canned ▪ fruit. For a special occasion, serve ▪ angel cake topped with fresh or canned unsweetened ▪ fruit and ▪ low-calorie dessert topping.

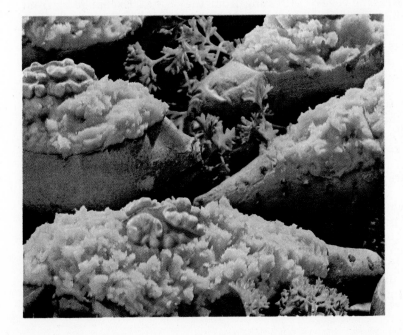

Your family will love twice-baked yams. Scoop out the yams and whip. Spoon back into the potato shells; heat through in oven. A ¼ cup serving equals ▪ 1 Bread Exchange. If butter is added and a walnut tops your serving, add ▪ Fat Exchanges. Accent with spices or herbs.

Vegetable exchanges

Serving ideas

- Add zest to vegetables by cooking with spices and herbs (see page 56). Start with ¼ teaspoon for each four servings; then taste before adding more.
- Top cooked vegetables with ■ pimiento, ■ chives, ■ grated cheese, or ■ croutons.
- Try cooking vegetables in ■ chicken broth or ■ beef broth.
- To complement ■ spinach, ■ broccoli, ■ Brussels sprouts, or ■ cabbage, serve ■ vinegar or a ■ lemon wedge.
- Have a glass of ■ tomato juice or ■ vegetable juice cocktail as an appetizer or snack. Dash in a squirt of ■ lemon juice, ■ Worcestershire sauce, or ■ seasoned salt and pepper for a pleasant change.
- Give ■ meats a delicious flavor by simmering in ■ tomato juice or canned ■ tomatoes along with ■ seasonings.
- Make tossed salads a real adventure. Try adding thinly sliced fresh ■ mushrooms, sliced ■ zucchini squash, or ■ cauliflowerets. Mix various kinds of ■ greens—escarole, endive, cabbage, spinach, Bibb lettuce, and Boston lettuce. Dress the salad with dressing from the ■ Fat Exchange or from the recipe section (page 56). You may use *1 tablespoon* of commercial low-calorie dressing containing less than 5 calories per *tablespoon* as a ■ Free Exchange.
- For relishes or snacks, remember ■ carrot curls, ■ celery sticks, ■ radish roses, and ■ cherry tomatoes.
- Vegetables also make attractive, tasty garnishes. Cut medium ■ tomatoes with a fancy sawtooth edge. Fill with ■ mushrooms or hot cooked vegetables. Broil a few minutes to heat through.
- On a cold wintery day serve homemade vegetable soup. Using ■ beef bouillon as the base, add ■ lean beef, ■ carrots, ■ peas, ■ tomatoes, ■ cabbage, and ■ seasonings. Before serving skim off excess fat.
- Skewer vegetables and broil alongside ■ meat or on a charcoal grill.
- Remember any butter on vegetables must be counted as a ■ Fat Exchange.

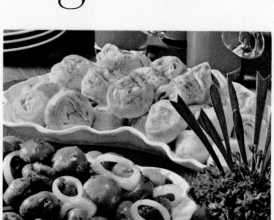

For tangy appetizers serve ■ Marinated Artichokes, ■ Pickled Mushrooms with onions, ■ Tomato Refresher (recipes on page 52).

Vegetable Exchanges are good in taste and loaded with other virtues. Yellow and green leafy kinds contain substances which the body converts into vitamin A. Some vegetables are rich in vitamin C, which is pretty skimpy in such fine foods as meats, milk, and cereals. (In the exchange listings * indicates rich sources of vitamin A and † indicates rich sources of vitamin C.) Vegetables have plenty of minerals too—iron for one.

They also contain cellulose which gives vegetables their structure. Cellulose is the indigestible part of plant foods which furnishes bulk in the intestinal tract and helps to maintain regularity.

You will note that there are two kinds of Vegetable Exchanges:

A. "As desired" vegetables which are very low in starch and calories, but good in vitamins, minerals, and satisfying bulk.

B. "Sturdy" vegetables which have more carbohydrate (and calories) in their makeup and a little protein too. As a result, you may substitute ◣ ½ Bread Exchange for ■ 1 Sturdy Vegetable Exchange.

Fruit exchange

Fruit Exchanges practically burst their flavor-buds for you! They're sweet by nature and don't need added sweetening, certainly not if one is watching calories. Just about all the calories in fruits come from carbohydrates, mostly fruit sugars, which are easy to digest and give quick energy.

Fruits in general have a laxative effect and keep us on the alkaline side, although they are acid when eaten. They're good mixers in salads, and unbeatable for eye-catching color. Fruits such as apricots, peaches, plums, raisins, have good iron content. Cantaloupe and some other fruits furnish surprising amounts of vitamin A. Fruits or their juices are the richest common sources of vitamin C, which is needed in relatively large daily amounts compared with other vitamins. Generally, the more acid the fruit, the richer the vitamin C content. Check high vitamin A and C foods in the exchange listings; include at least one of each in the diet everyday.

Serving ideas

• Use either *fresh* ■ fruits and juices or canned *unsweetened* (water-pack) or artificially sweetened ■ fruits (usually called "dietetic-pack" and located in a special diet section at the market.) Read labels carefully.
• For breakfast you may prefer an ■ orange juice ritual or a wide variety of ■ fruits such as: grapefruit half; banana, berries, or peaches on ■ cereal; plumped raisins on ■ hot cereal; baked apple; melon wedge; or mixed fruit cup.
• Appetizers might be ■ fruit juice, ■ melon wedge with ■ lemon slice, ■ papaya with ■ lime wedge, ■ melon balls, or ■ peach half filled with berries.
• Salads are limited only by imagination— ■ fruit arranged with ■ cottage cheese and ■ ham roll-ups; ■ fruits molded in ■ low-calorie gelatin; ■ prunes, ■ peaches, or pears stuffed with ■ cream cheese; or chicken salad on ■ pineapple rings.
• ■ Fruits bring a sweet ending to a meal in the form of: fresh fruit and ■ cheese tray, fruit spooned over ■ sherbet, canned fruit and juice, broiled grapefruit, or fresh or canned unsweetened fruit combinations. For many luscious fruit desserts, see the recipe section on pages 68-71.
• If you are a real fruit lover, occasionally substitute ■ ▲ 1½ Fruit Exchanges for ■ 1 Bread Exchange. This will allow you to enjoy a glorious fruit plate.
• Fruits make attractive, meant-to-be eaten garnishes too. Bright grape clusters, orange cartwheels, apple rings, pineapple twists, and fresh cherries with stems double as garnishes and ■ Fruit Exchanges.
• Fruits make an ideal between-meal snack — ■ apples, ■ oranges—you name it.

As an appetizer, a salad, or a dessert, the tart punch of this ■ Green 'n Gold Compote will brighten your meal. (See page 69 for recipe.)

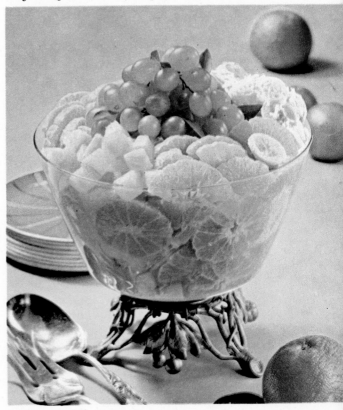

Milk exchange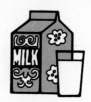

Milk is a major source of calcium, phosphorus, and riboflavin in the average American diet. Its protein is top quality, its carbohydrates easily assimilated by babies. About half of the calories of whole milk are accounted for by fat, which is removed from skim milk, buttermilk, or nonfat dry milk solids. All that is lost, besides calories reducers won't miss, are fat-soluble vitamins A and D. Thus, the Milk Exchange is based on skim milk. In equal volume, skim milk contains a little more protein, minerals, and water-soluble vitamins than whole milk. Milk Exchanges don't have to be drunk. They can be used in cooking, on cereals, or in desserts.

Serving ideas

• One ▉ Milk Exchange is 8 ounces of skim milk, buttermilk, or beverage made from instant nonfat dry milk.

• If you'd rather drink 8 ounces of ▉ whole milk, you can reduce it to ▉ 1 Milk Exchange by omitting ▉ 2 Fat Exchanges from your diet. Most people prefer to drink ▉ skim milk and use the ▉ 2 Fat Exchanges elsewhere in their menu.
• Milk with 2% butterfat equals ▉ 1 Milk Exchange plus ▉ 1 Fat Exchange. Some people find this modification more palatable.
• Plain yogurt rates the same as whole milk. One cup of yogurt equals ▉ 1 Milk Exchange plus ▉ 2 Fat Exchanges. Yogurt forms the base for pleasant salad dressings and fruit dress-ups.
• Four ounces of evaporated *skim* milk is equal to ▉ 1 Milk Exchange. To add variety, whip and use as a topping for fruit. See page 71 for recipe.
• Do you drink several cups of ▉ coffee a day? If you add milk, remember to count it as ▉ Milk Exchanges.

Fat exchange

Fats are the sliest food exchanges. They pack lots of calories into deceptively small packages. And they taste so good, add so much to the deliciousness of other foods. Fats are often "hidden" in foods we like best, causing a pile up around the waistline before we know it.

Fats and oils give us essential fatty acids, calories, some fat-soluble vitamins, and nothing else of much significance. But if you don't let them run away with you, they're great friends, not enemies. Fats slow the emptying time of the stomach, ward off hunger sensations, provide energy, and are needed for healthy skin, hair, and membranes.

Serving ideas

• Note that ▉ 1 Fat Exchange equals 1 *measuring teaspoon* of butter, margarine, shortening, or salad oil.

• The ▉ cream family (heavy, light, sour) counts as ▉ Fat Exchanges. Instead of cream in your coffee, try ▉ skim milk—just use more than the usual amount of cream. One tablespoon of heavy cream is equal to 2 tablespoons whipped cream; or try ▉ low-calorie dessert topping mix (see page 31).
• Non-stick surfaced pans allow you to cook without fat—use ▉ Fat Exchanges elsewhere to add variety to your meals.
• ▉ Crisp bacon is delicious crumbled atop hot cooked vegetables, ▉ baked potato, or vegetable salad.
• ▉ Olives and ▉ avocados add an unusual flair to sandwiches and salads.
• ▉ Nuts are great for between-meal snacks or atop vegetables or as a garnish on puddings and other desserts.
• Stuff various ▉ fruits with ▉ cream cheese whipped with a little ▉ skim milk for attractive, tasty salads or desserts.

Free exchange

The only limit on Free Exchanges is your capacity. They're insignificant as far as calories go, but they add savors and flavors and gourmet touches that make meals delightful to serve and eat.

Serving ideas

• ■ Lemon adds tang to ■ broccoli, ■ Brussels sprouts, and ■ spinach. It's great in refreshing drinks such as ■ lemonade (recipe on page 72) or ■ iced tea.

• ■ Rhubarb Sauce makes a delightful tart ending to a meal (recipe on page 70).

• ■ Tea and ■ coffee are favorites to sip as you work along. Add ■ non-caloric sweetener, ■ skim milk, or ■ cream according to your Daily Meal Plan.

• ■ Broth or ■ bouillon serves as a pick-me-up snack, as cooking liquid for ■ meats and vegetables, and as a base for soups.

• ■ Unflavored gelatin and ■ low-calorie gelatin make luscious molded salads and chilled desserts.

• Sour or unsweetened ■ dill pickles are tasty meal accompaniments—also add pleasant flavor and crunch to meat sandwiches.

• ■ Non-caloric sweetener should be used in moderate amounts in place of sugar. It is available in liquid, tablet, and powdered form.

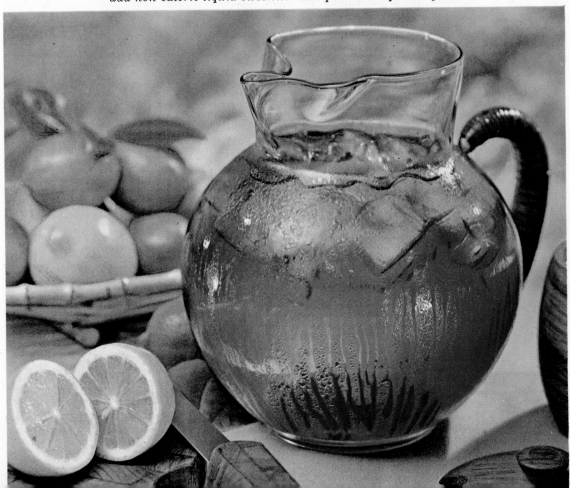

Working hard and need a break? Relax with cool refreshing iced tea, accented with tangy lemon or lime. For a sweet touch add non-caloric liquid sweetener and pour over sparkling ice.

Alcohol slows progress

No matter what wishful thinkers say, alcohol calories count the same as others. In fact, alcohol packs a bigger caloric punch than protein and carbohydrate, and nearly as much as fat. So weight watchers beware!

It is true that alcohol calories can't be stored in the form of fat body tissue. They are burned (oxidized) quite promptly. The catch is that while alcohol calories are burning, the calories of other foods are available for storage as fat body tissue if total caloric intake is in excess of needs. So reducers who ingest alcohol calories have to take them into account in their diet.

A balanced low-calorie reducing diet furnishes essential nutrients. Therefore, foods should never be subtracted from a reducing diet to "make room for" alcohol calories. The calories of an alcoholic beverage should be *added to* the calories of a reducing diet. This slows the speed of the reducing diet to the extent of the added calories.

It is easy to figure the calorie values of whiskey, rum, vodka, and similar "hard" liquors taken straight or with water. Labels on the bottles give the "proof" of the liquor; for instance, 86-proof or 100-proof. *One ounce* of such liquor contains as many calories as its proof. For example, one ounce of 100-proof liquor contains 100 calories.

Mixed drinks with added ingredients such as ginger ale or fruit juices have calories in addition to alcohol calories. Bar sugar counts the same as table sugar. However, carbonated water is a Free Exchange.

For practical purposes relevant to reducing, the caloric charge of representative alcoholic beverages can be compared to approximate caloric equivalents from the "luxury" Fat Exchanges.

ALCOHOL CALORIES COUNT TOO

BEVERAGE WITH SERVING AMOUNT	APPROXIMATELY EQUIVALENT IN CALORIES TO:
Martini, 3½ ounces	3 teaspoons mayonnaise
Manhattan, 3½ ounces	4 tablespoons French dressing
Champagne cocktail, 4 ounces	4 tablespoons coffee cream
Highball with water, 8 ounces	4 slices bacon
with ginger ale, 8 ounces	5 slices bacon
Glass of beer, 8 ounces	15 small peanuts
Dinner wine, dry, 3½ ounces	2 teaspoons butter
Dessert wine, fortified, sweet, 3½ ounces	⅓ avocado, 4-inch diameter
Daiquiri, 3½ ounces	3 tablespoons cream cheese
Old Fashioned, 4 ounces	4 tablespoons sour cream
Tom Collins, 10 ounces	4 tablespoons whipping cream

Menu planning steps

When there are no calories to count, menu planning can be fun. The Daily Meal Plans (1000, 1200, or 1500 calories) on page 27 and the Exchange Lists on pages 28-31 are the working tools for menu planning.

Decide on the Daily Meal Plan which will allow you to lose not more than 2 pounds a week. This Daily Meal Plan is your guide to menu planning. Make your selections as your menu guide directs from the exchange lists.

The following 7 Menu Planning Steps will assist you in making the selections:

1. Choose the main dish based on the ▓ Meat Exchanges.
2. Select ▓ Bread Exchanges to accompany the main dish.
3. Pick compatible ▓ As Desired Vegetable Exchanges and ▓ Sturdy Vegetable Exchange if allowed.
4. Decide on a ▓ Fruit Exchange for salad, appetizer, or dessert.
5. Include ▓ Milk Exchanges not used in cooking as a beverage.
6. Include ▓ Fat Exchanges not used in cooking.
7. Add ▓ Free Exchanges to round out the meal.

For example, to plan a 1500 calorie dinner, first consult the 1500 Calorie Daily Meal Plan which is given below.

DINNER

▓ ▓ ▓ 3 Meat Exchanges
▓ ▓ 2 Bread Exchanges
▓ As Desired Vegetable Exchange
▓ 1 Sturdy Vegetable Exchange
▓ 1 Fruit Exchange
◣ ½ Milk Exchange
▓ 2 Fat Exchanges
▓ Free Exchanges

Then follow the 7 Menu Planning Steps:

1. Main dish—According to the daily meal plan, ▓ ▓ ▓ 3 Meat Exchanges are allowed at dinner. One serving of Deviled Swiss Steak* (*indicates see recipe section) equals ▓ ▓ ▓ 3 Meat Exchanges.
2. Bread— ▓ ▓ 2 Bread Exchanges are allowed. A baked potato, ▓ 1 Bread Exchange, goes well with steak. The other Bread Exchange is lemon sherbet for dessert.
3. Vegetable—A crisp vegetable salad qualifies as an ▓ As Desired Vegetable Exchange. Green peas have an exchange value of ▓ 1 Sturdy Vegetable Exchange.
4. Fruit—Utilize ▓ 1 Fruit Exchange for appetizer or dessert since tossed salad is already on the menu. How about fresh or unsweetened frozen strawberries over the lemon sherbet to make a sundae?
5. Milk— ◣ ½ Milk Exchange should be consumed. Since no milk was used in cooking, drink 4 ounces with meal.
6. Fat— ▓ ▓ 2 Fat Exchanges are allowed. Use ▓ 1 Fat Exchange as 1 teaspoon butter or margarine on the green peas. Use the other ▓ Fat Exchange as 1 teaspoon butter on the ▓ baked potato.
7. Free Exchanges—To complete the meal add ▓ tea or ▓ coffee and 2 tablespoons ▓ Slim-trim Dressing* for the salad.

1500 CALORIE DINNER MENU

▓ ▓ ▓ Deviled Swiss Steak*
▓ 1 small Baked Potato with
▓ 1 teaspoon Butter
▓ Tossed Vegetable Salad with
▓ Slim-trim Dressing*
▓ ½ cup Green Peas with
▓ 1 teaspoon Butter
▓ ⅓ cup Lemon Sherbet with
▓ 1 cup Strawberries
◣ 4 ounces Skim Milk
▓ Coffee or Tea

In planning your own menus, make your choices according to personal taste, foods in season, or what you happen to have on hand. To add variety to your menus use recipes on pages 52-73. The exchange value of one serving is given in each recipe.

Sample menus on the following pages will help you compare meal plans, menus, and the exchanges. Read the meal plans and menus till you understand how they fit together.

*See recipe section.

1000 calorie menus

A daily intake of 1000 calories is the minimum level most doctors recommend without close medical supervision. Check to make sure you will not lose more than 2 pounds a week on this caloric level.

The sample menus on pages 41-51 will help you compare meal plans, menus, and exchanges. Food items marked by * on menus are from the recipe section. For each recipe the exchange value of 1 serving is given for your convenience.

To compare the meal plans and the menus, follow the 7 Menu Planning Steps:

1. Choose the main dish based on the ■ Meat Exchanges.
2. Select ■ Bread Exchanges to accompany the main dish.
3. Pick compatible ■ As Desired Vegetable Exchanges and ■ Sturdy Vegetable Exchange according to your meal plan.
4. Decide on a ■ Fruit Exchange for salad, appetizer, or dessert.
5. Include ■ Milk Exchanges not used in cooking as a beverage.
6. Include ■ Fat Exchanges not used in cooking.
7. Add ■ Free Exchanges to round out the meal.

When comparing the menus with the Daily Meal Plan, you will discover some menus use extra exchanges and some are missing an exchange or two—they have simply been moved from one meal to another. To trace these moving exchanges, two headings have been used: Exchanges Not Used and Extra Exchanges Used. Remember in weight reduction it is the *total* daily intake that is important. Therefore, the daily total of Extra Exchanges Used should equal Exchanges Not Used.

A complete discussion of each menu can be found under Exchange Tips. Compare the Daily Meal Plan and the menus until you understand how they fit together. Then plan your own menus.

DAILY MEAL PLAN

BREAKFAST

■ *1 Meat Exchange*
■ *1 Bread Exchange*
■ *As Desired Vegetable*
■ *1 Fruit Exchange*
◣ *½ Milk Exchange*
■ *1 Fat Exchange*
■ *Free Exchanges*

LUNCH

■■■ *3 Meat Exchanges*
■ *As Desired Vegetable*
■ *1 Fruit Exchange*
■ *1 Milk Exchange*
■ *Free Exchanges*

DINNER

■■■ *3 Meat Exchanges*
■ *As Desired Vegetable*
■ *1 Sturdy Vegetable*
■ *1 Fruit Exchange*
◣ *½ Milk Exchange*
■ *Free Exchanges*

BREAKFAST

- ■ *1 Egg, fried in non-stick pan*
- ■ *1 Baking-powder Biscuit*
- ■ *1 teaspoon Butter*
- ■ *½ cup Tomato Juice*
- ◣ *½ cup Skim Milk*
- ■ *Coffee*

MIDMORNING SNACK

- ■ *Spiced Pineapple Sparkle**

LUNCH

- ■■■■ *Chef's Salad* with*
  ■ *Gourmet Dressing**
- ■ *Plum Whip**
- ■ *1 cup Skim Milk*

DINNER

- ■■■ *Pampered Beef Fillets**
- ■ *Cauliflowerets with*
  ■ *Slim-trim Dressing**
- ◣ *¼ cup Green Peas and Onions*
- ◣ *¼ cup Parslied Carrots*
- ■ *Rainbow Melon Julep**
- ◣ *½ cup Skim Milk*
- ■ *Coffee or Tea*

*see recipe section

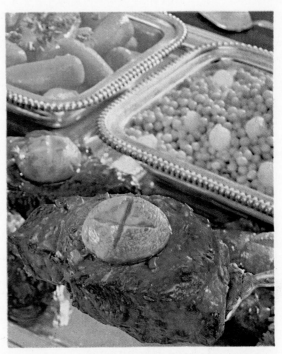

For an elegant meal serve Pampered Beef Fillets with fresh mushroom crowns atop. Green peas and onions and parslied carrots complement the meat and add color.

✳ EXCHANGE TIPS

Try frying an egg in a non-stick pan to save the fat for a baking-powder biscuit. Simply place an egg in the skillet and cook to desired degree of doneness.

A midmorning snack will help keep those hunger pangs away. Try saving a ■ Fruit Exchange (or any exchange you desire) from your breakfast menu and treat yourself to a refreshing midmorning break.

Lunch looks small? Be careful, your eyes may be deceiving you. Chef's Salad is quite filling and good to the last crunch when topped with Gourmet Dressing. By using a salad dressing from the ■ Free Exchange you can have each mouthful of salad nicely coated with dressing.

Dinner is your largest meal. Eat slowly and savor every bite. In order to have a serving *each* of carrots and peas, simply divide your ½ cup serving into two ¼-cup servings. This is a trick to remember when you are eating out, too.

DAILY MEAL PLAN

BREAKFAST

- 1 Meat Exchange
- 1 Bread Exchange
- As Desired Vegetable
- 1 Fruit Exchange
- ½ Milk Exchange
- 1 Fat Exchange
- Free Exchanges

LUNCH

- 3 Meat Exchanges
- As Desired Vegetable
- 1 Fruit Exchange
- 1 Milk Exchange
- Free Exchanges

DINNER

- 3 Meat Exchanges
- As Desired Vegetable
- 1 Sturdy Vegetable
- 1 Fruit Exchange
- ½ Milk Exchange
- Free Exchanges

BREAKFAST

- ¾ cup Dry Cereal with
  ½ cup Skim Milk
- ½ cup Orange Juice
- Coffee

EXCHANGES NOT USED
- 1 Meat Exchange
- 1 Fat Exchange

LUNCH

Jiffy Chicken Soup:
- 3 ounces cooked chicken
  in chicken consomme

Pear-Cottage Cheese Salad:
- 2 small dietetic-pack
  pear halves
- ¼ cup cottage cheese
- lettuce cup
- 1 tablespoon French
  salad dressing

- Rhubarb Sauce*
- 1 cup Skim Milk

EXTRA EXCHANGES USED
- 1 Meat Exchange
- 1 Fat Exchange

DINNER

- Lamb Chop Oriental*
- Asparagus Spears
- ½ cup Winter Squash

Apple Raisin Salad:
- ½ small apple
- 1 tablespoon raisins

- Coffee Chiffon*
- Coffee or Tea

*see recipe section

✳ EXCHANGE TIPS

The ■ As Desired Vegetable Exchange was included at breakfast to provide the option of tomato juice or vegetable juice. In this way you could *save*, not omit, the ■ 1 Fruit Exchange for a midmorning snack. The ■ 1 Fat Exchange not used at breakfast is used at lunch for salad dressing.

The ■ 1 Meat Exchange normally eaten at breakfast is added to the lunch menu. Three ounces of chicken used in the Jiffy Chicken Soup equals ■ ■ ■ 3 Meat Exchanges—the amount listed in the Daily Meal Plan for lunch. However, ¼ cup cottage cheese is used in the salad adding ■ 1 Meat Exchange. As a result, for lunch you have a total of ■ ■ ■ ■ 4 Meat Exchanges, borrowing the extra exchange from breakfast—Exchanges Not Used at breakfast equal Extra Exchanges Used at lunch.

In the dinner menu the ■ 1 Fruit Exchange was divided into 2 one-half Fruit Exchanges (◣ + ◣ = ■ 1 Fruit Exchange) to add variety to the salad.

✳ EXCHANGE TIPS

Remember it is not necessary to include an ■ As Desired Vegetable Exchange at breakfast. Other exchanges not used at breakfast are ■ 1 Bread Exchange and ▨ 1 Fat Exchange.

With a daily intake of 1000 calories, ■ 1 Bread Exchange and ▨ 1 Fat Exchange must be saved from breakfast in order to have a sandwich for lunch.

To measure the amount of skim milk used on cereal or fruit, such as Peaches and Milk, pour the skim milk into a measuring cup; then pour the desired amount over the fruit. You can either drink the remaining milk or you can save it for supper or late evening snack as is shown in this menu.

In comparing the exchanges, the Exchanges Not Used at breakfast equal the Extra Exchanges Used at lunch. The Exchange Not Used at lunch equals the Extra Exchange Used at dinner.

As you can see, the variety in daily menus is limited only by your imagination.

BREAKFAST

- ■ 1 Egg Omelet, cooked in non-stick pan
- ■ ¼ Cantaloupe
- ◣ ½ cup Skim Milk
- ■ Coffee

EXCHANGES NOT USED

- ■ 1 Bread Exchange
- ▨ 1 Fat Exchange

LUNCH

Bologna Cheese Sandwich:
- ■ ■ 2 slices Bologna
- ■ 1 slice American cheese
- ■ 1 slice bread
- ▨ 1 teaspoon butter

- ■ Sliced Tomatoes

Peaches and Milk:
- ■ 1 medium peach, sliced
- ◣ ½ cup skim milk

EXTRA EXCHANGES USED

- ■ 1 Bread Exchange
- ▨ 1 Fat Exchange

EXCHANGES NOT USED

- ◣ ½ Milk Exchange

DINNER

- ▨ Jamaican Swizzle*
- ■ ■ ■ 3 ounces Baked Chicken
- ■ French-style Green Beans
- ▨ ½ cup Beets and Onion Rings
- ■ Green 'n Gold Compote*
- ■ 1 cup Skim Milk
- ■ Coffee or Tea

EXTRA EXCHANGES USED

- ◣ ½ Milk Exchange

*see recipe section

1200 calorie menus

More calories, increased selections, greater variety—these are the advantages of choosing a daily intake of 1200 calories. Your reducing speed may be slower, but your eating satisfaction will be greater.

The sample menus on pages 41-51 will help you compare meal plans, menus, and exchanges. Food items marked by * on menus are from the recipe section. For each recipe the exchange value of 1 serving is given for your convenience.

To compare the meal plans and the menus, follow the 7 Menu Planning Steps:

1. Choose the main dish based on the ■ Meat Exchanges.
2. Select ■ Bread Exchanges to accompany the main dish.
3. Pick compatible ■ As Desired Vegetable Exchanges and ■ Sturdy Vegetable Exchange according to your meal plan.
4. Decide on a ■ Fruit Exchange for salad, appetizer, or dessert.
5. Include ■ Milk Exchanges not used in cooking as a beverage.
6. Include ■ Fat Exchanges not used in cooking.
7. Add ■ Free Exchanges to round out the meal.

When comparing the menus with the Daily Meal Plan, you will discover some menus use extra exchanges and some are missing an exchange or two—they have simply been moved from one meal to another. To trace these moving exchanges, two headings have been used: Exchanges Not Used and Extra Exchanges Used. Remember in weight reduction it is the *total* daily intake that is important. Therefore, the daily total of Extra Exchanges Used should equal Exchanges Not Used.

A complete discussion of each menu can be found under Exchange Tips. Compare the Daily Meal Plan and the menus until you understand how they fit together. Then plan your own menus.

DAILY MEAL PLAN

BREAKFAST

■ *1 Meat Exchange*
■ *1 Bread Exchange*
■ *As Desired Vegetable*
■ *1 Fruit Exchange*
◤ *½ Milk Exchange*
■ *1 Fat Exchange*
■ *Free Exchanges*

LUNCH

■■■ *3 Meat Exchanges*
■ *1 Bread Exchange*
■ *As Desired Vegetable*
■ *1 Fruit Exchange*
■ *1 Milk Exchange*
■ *1 Fat Exchange*
■ *Free Exchanges*

DINNER

■■■ *3 Meat Exchanges*
■ *1 Bread Exchange*
■ *As Desired Vegetable*
■ *1 Sturdy Vegetable*
■ *1 Fruit Exchange*
◤ *½ Milk Exchange*
■ *1 Fat Exchange*
■ *Free Exchanges*

BREAKFAST

- 1 Soft Boiled Egg
- 1 Slice Toast with
     1 teaspoon Butter
- ½ cup Orange Juice
- ½ cup Skim Milk
- Coffee

LUNCH

Skilletburgers*

Peach Salad:
     lettuce slice
     2 dietetic-pack
          peach halves
     low-calorie French
          salad dressing

Baked Custard*
Coffee or Tea

EXTRA EXCHANGES USED
1 Sturdy Vegetable
     Exchange

EXCHANGES NOT USED
½ Milk Exchange

DINNER

Barbecued Pork and Beans*

Crookneck Squash with
     ½ teaspoon Butter

Cabbage Pineapple Slaw*
⅔ cup Chocolate-flavored
     Low-calorie Pudding
Iced Tea

EXTRA EXCHANGES USED
½ Milk Exchange

EXCHANGES NOT USED
1 Sturdy Vegetable
     Exchange

*see recipe section

EXCHANGE TIPS

One serving of a mixed dish often provides many different exchanges; however, it may not provide the exact amount of each exchange needed for a particular menu. For example, 1 serving of Skilletburgers equals 2 Meat Exchanges, but 3 Meat Exchanges are needed for lunch. By adding 1 serving of Baked Custard which equals 1 Meat Exchange, the two servings total 3 Meat Exchanges. However, in order to serve Skilletburgers at lunch, 1 Sturdy Vegetable Exchange must be moved from the dinner menu to the lunch menu. The Baked Custard has only ½ Milk Exchange. The unused ½ Milk Exchange is added to the ½ Milk Exchange at dinner to equal 1 Milk Exchange—perfect for Chocolate-flavored Low-calorie Pudding.

The low-calorie French salad dressing used at lunch is commercially bottled.

Going to a potluck or a family reunion? Take Barbecued Pork and Beans topped with an onion and a lemon slice. Everyone will rave and no one will know your secret.

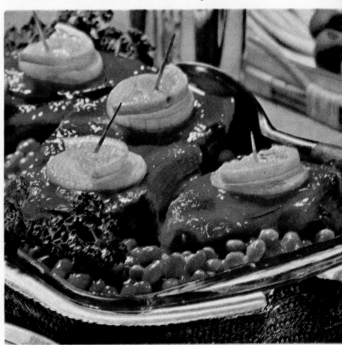

DAILY MEAL PLAN

BREAKFAST

- 1 Meat Exchange
- 1 Bread Exchange
- As Desired Vegetable
- 1 Fruit Exchange
- ½ Milk Exchange
- 1 Fat Exchange
- Free Exchanges

LUNCH

- 3 Meat Exchanges
- 1 Bread Exchange
- As Desired Vegetable
- 1 Fruit Exchange
- 1 Milk Exchange
- 1 Fat Exchange
- Free Exchanges

DINNER

- 3 Meat Exchanges
- 1 Bread Exchange
- As Desired Vegetable
- 1 Sturdy Vegetable
- 1 Fruit Exchange
- ½ Milk Exchange
- 1 Fat Exchange
- Free Exchanges

BREAKFAST

Broiled Cheese Toast:
- 1 slice American cheese
- 1 slice bread
- 1 teaspoon butter
- 1 Orange, sectioned
- 1 cup Skim Milk
- Coffee

EXTRA EXCHANGES USED

- ½ Milk Exchange

LUNCH

- Cream of Asparagus Soup
- Broiled Veal Chop
- Broiled Tomato* with
    1 tablespoon Sour Cream
- Lime-applesauce Mold*
- 1 cup Skim Milk
- Tea

DINNER

- Poached Salmon* with
    Cucumber-dill Sauce*
- 1 small Baked Potato
- Crisp Green Salad with
    Low-calorie Italian Salad
    Dressing and
    ½ cup Croutons
- Creamy Apricot Dessert:
    4 dietetic-pack apricot
    halves
    2½ tablespoons dessert
    topping mix
- Coffee or Tea

EXCHANGES NOT USED

- ½ Milk Exchange

*see recipe section

✻ EXCHANGE TIPS

For breakfast it isn't necessary to eat an ■ As Desired Vegetable Exchange. This exchange was included at breakfast to provide the option of tomato juice or vegetable juice cocktail. In this way you could *save*, not omit, the ■ 1 Fruit Exchange for a midmorning snack.

If you enjoy drinking a glass of milk with breakfast, add the ◣ ½ Milk Exchange from dinner to the breakfast menu.

On a cold winter day, a bowl of soup at lunch is a hearty addition to the menu. One half can of condensed cream of asparagus soup made with water equals ■ 1 Bread Exchange (see page 31).

Remember ■ 1 Sturdy Vegetable Exchange can be substituted for ◣ ½ Bread Exchange. For example, in the dinner menu, croutons, normally ◣ ½ Bread Exchange, were used as ■ 1 Sturdy Vegetable Exchange. The low-calorie Italian salad dressing is the commercially bottled salad dressing with less than 5 calories per tablespoon.

✻ EXCHANGE TIPS

One egg fried in a small skillet with 1 teaspoon of melted butter equals ■ 1 Meat Exchange and ▨ 1 Fat Exchange. When served with a buttered English muffin, ▨ ▨ 2 Fat Exchanges are used at breakfast. This requires shifting ■ 1 Fat Exchange from lunch to breakfast. If the egg is fried in a non-stick pan, no shortening or butter is used. Consequently, no shifting of Fat Exchanges would be necessary.

In order to include carrot curls on the relish plate at noon the ◣ ½ Sturdy Vegetable Exchange must be transferred from dinner to lunch, still leaving ◣ ½ Sturdy Vegetable Exchange at dinner. The ■ 1 Fruit Exchange normally eaten at lunch was saved for a midafternoon snack.

For the traditional Thanksgiving dinner, serve Roast Turkey with Bread Stuffing. One ■ Bread Exchange at dinner requires a choice of either Bread Stuffing or mashed potatoes. To prepare Herbed Onions refer to Vegetable Seasoning Guide on page 56.

BREAKFAST

- ■ *1 Egg, fried in*
  ▨ *1 teaspoon Butter*
- ▨ *½ English Muffin with*
  ▨ *1 teaspoon Butter*
- ■ *1 cup Raspberries with*
  ◣ *½ cup Skim Milk*
- ■ *Coffee*

EXTRA EXCHANGES USED
■ *1 Fat Exchange*

LUNCH

- ■ ■ ■ *No Crust Pizza**
  Relish Plate:
  ■ *As Desired Vegetables*
  ◣ *¼ cup carrot curls*
- ▨ *⅓ cup Pineapple Sherbet*
- ■ *1 cup Skim Milk*

EXTRA EXCHANGES USED
◣ *½ Sturdy Vegetable*

EXCHANGES NOT USED
▨ *1 Fat Exchange*

MIDAFTERNOON SNACK
■ *1 small Apple*

DINNER

- ■ ■ ■ *3 ounces Roast Turkey*
  ⅓ cup Bread Stuffing or*
  ▨ *½ cup Mashed Potatoes*
- ■ *Buttered Green Beans with*
  1 teaspoon Butter
- ◣ *¼ cup Herbed Onions*
- ◣ *Molded Cranberry*
  *Waldorfs**
- ◣ *Tapioca Pudding* with*
  ◣ *½ cup Strawberries*
- ■ *Coffee or Tea*

EXCHANGES NOT USED
◣ *½ Sturdy Vegetable*

*see recipe section

1500 calorie menus

A daily intake of 1500 calories can fill your meals with hearty dishes and cause hunger pangs to vanish. Menu ideas are limited only by the imagination of the cook.

The sample menus on pages 41-51 will help you compare meal plans, menus, and exchanges. Food items marked by * on menus are from the recipe section. For each recipe, the exchange value of one serving is given for your convenience.

To compare the meal plans and the menus, follow the 7 Menu Planning Steps:

1. Choose the main dish based on the ■ Meat Exchanges.
2. Select ■ Bread Exchanges to accompany the main dish.
3. Pick compatible ■ As Desired Vegetable Exchanges and ■ Sturdy Vegetable Exchange according to your meal plan.
4. Decide on a ■ Fruit Exchange for salad, appetizer, or dessert.
5. Include ■ Milk Exchanges not used in cooking as a beverage.
6. Include ■ Fat Exchanges not used in cooking.
7. Add ■ Free Exchanges to round out the meal.

When comparing the menus with the Daily Meal Plan, you will notice that some menus use extra exchanges and some are missing an exchange or two—they have simply been moved from one meal to another. To trace these moving exchanges, two headings have been used: Exchanges Not Used and Extra Exchanges Used. Remember, in weight reduction it is the *total* daily intake that is important. Therefore, the daily total of Extra Exchanges Used should equal Exchanges Not Used.

A complete discussion of each menu can be found under Exchange Tips. Compare the Daily Meal Plan and the menus until you understand how they fit together. Then plan your own menus.

DAILY MEAL PLAN

BREAKFAST

- ■ 1 Meat Exchange
- ■ 1 Bread Exchange
- ■ As Desired Vegetable
- ■ 1 Fruit Exchange
- ◣ ½ Milk Exchange
- ■ ■ 2 Fat Exchanges
- ■ Free Exchanges

LUNCH

- ■ ■ ■ 3 Meat Exchanges
- ■ ■ 2 Bread Exchanges
- ■ As Desired Vegetable
- ■ 1 Fruit Exchange
- ■ 1 Milk Exchange
- ■ ■ 2 Fat Exchanges
- ■ Free Exchanges

DINNER

- ■ ■ ■ 3 Meat Exchanges
- ■ ■ 2 Bread Exchanges
- ■ As Desired Vegetable
- ■ 1 Sturdy Vegetable
- ■ 1 Fruit Exchange
- ◣ ½ Milk Exchange
- ■ ■ 2 Fat Exchanges
- ■ Free Exchanges

BREAKFAST

- ■ *1 Egg, scrambled with*
- ◣ *½ ounce Breakfast Ham*
- ■ *1 slice Toast with*
- □ *1 teaspoon Butter*

Banana and Milk:
- □ *½ small banana*
- ◣ *½ cup skim milk*
- ▨ *Coffee*

EXTRA EXCHANGES USED
- ◣ *½ Meat Exchange*

EXCHANGES NOT USED
- □ *1 Fat Exchange*

LUNCH

Roast Beef Sandwich:
- ■■■ *3 ounces beef*
- ■■ *2 slices bread*
- □□ *2 teaspoons butter*

Asparagus Salad:
- ■ *asparagus and lettuce*
- □ *1 tablespoon French salad dressing*
- ■ *Ruby Fruit Compote**
- ■ *1 cup Skim Milk*

EXTRA EXCHANGES USED
- □ *1 Fat Exchange*

DINNER

- ▨ *Pineapple Passion**
- ■■■◣ *Skillet Spaghetti**
- ■□
- ■ *1 slice French Bread with*
- □ *1 teaspoon Butter*
- ■ *Crisp Green Salad with*
- ▨ *Low-calorie Italian Salad Dressing*
- ▨◣ *Ribbon Fudge Parfait**
- ■ *Coffee or Tea*

EXCHANGES NOT USED
- ◣ *½ Meat Exchange*

* See recipe section

EXCHANGE TIPS

One serving of a mixed dish often leaves a fraction of an exchange unused. For example, at dinner one serving of Skillet Spaghetti served without added Parmesan cheese equals ■ ■ ◣ 2½ Meat Exchanges. This leaves ◣ ½ Meat Exchange to be eaten at another meal—breakfast. Combine ½ ounce of ham and 1 scrambled egg for a total of ■ ◣ 1½ Meat Exchanges.

By saving □ 1 Fat Exchange from breakfast, a total of □ □ □ 3 Fat Exchanges can be used at lunch. If you are planning to serve a sandwich, both slices of bread can be buttered and there is an additional □ 1 Fat Exchange left for salad dressing.

Caution: there are two listings for French salad dressing. One tablespoon of regular French salad dressing (page 29) equals □ 1 Fat Exchange. The commercially bottled French salad dressing with less than five calories per tablespoon (see Packaged Exchanges, page 31) is a ▨ Free Exchange.

For an informal dinner, everyone will enjoy Skillet Spaghetti served hot at the table. If topped with three tablespoons Parmesan cheese add ◣ ½ Meat Exchange.

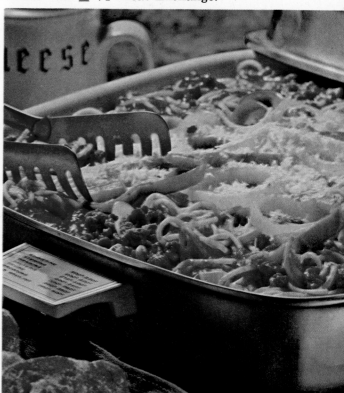

DAILY MEAL PLAN

BREAKFAST

- ■ 1 Meat Exchange
- ■ 1 Bread Exchange
- ■ As Desired Vegetable
- ■ 1 Fruit Exchange
- ◣ ½ Milk Exchange
- ■ ■ 2 Fat Exchanges
- ■ Free Exchanges

LUNCH

- ■ ■ ■ 3 Meat Exchanges
- ■ ■ 2 Bread Exchanges
- ■ As Desired Vegetable
- ■ 1 Fruit Exchange
- ■ 1 Milk Exchange
- ■ ■ 2 Fat Exchanges
- ■ Free Exchanges

DINNER

- ■ ■ ■ 3 Meat Exchanges
- ■ ■ 2 Bread Exchanges
- ■ As Desired Vegetable
- ■ 1 Sturdy Vegetable
- ■ 1 Fruit Exchange
- ◣ ½ Milk Exchange
- ■ ■ 2 Fat Exchanges
- ■ Free Exchanges

BREAKFAST

- ■ ½ cup Oatmeal with
- ■   2 tablespoons Raisins
- ◣ ½ cup Skim Milk
- ■ Coffee

EXCHANGES NOT USED

- ■ 1 Meat Exchange
- ■ ■ 2 Fat Exchanges

LUNCH

- ■ ■ ■ ■ ■ ■ Peachy Ham Swisser*
- ■ Perfection Salad* with
    2 tablespoons Low-calorie
    Mayonnaise
- ■ ■ ■ ½ cup Vanilla Ice Cream
- ◣ ½ cup Skim Milk

EXTRA EXCHANGES USED

- ■ ■ 2 Fat Exchanges

EXCHANGES NOT USED

- ◣ ½ Milk Exchange

DINNER

- ■ Tomato Juice with
- ■   3 Shredded Wheat Wafers
- ■ ■ ■ ■ French Herbed Chicken*
- ■ ½ cup Rice with
- ■   1 teaspoon Butter

  Apple Pinwheel Salad:
- ■   1 small apple, sliced
- ■   lettuce leaf
- ■   1 tablespoon French
      salad dressing
- ■ ⅔ cup Butterscotch Low-
      calorie Pudding
- ■ Coffee or Tea

EXTRA EXCHANGES USED

- ■ 1 Meat Exchange
- ◣ ½ Milk Exchange

* see recipe section

✳ EXCHANGE TIPS

An appealing small breakfast can make larger noon and evening meals possible. For example, at breakfast ■ 1 Meat Exchange and ■ ■ 2 Fat Exchanges were not used. The ■ 1 Meat Exchange was transferred to the dinner menu allowing 1 serving of French Herbed Chicken. The ■ ■ 2 Fat Exchanges were shifted to the lunch menu totaling ■ ■ ■ ■ 4 Fat Exchanges.

By saving ■ ■ 2 Fat Exchanges at breakfast, ½ cup ice cream equaling ■ 1 Bread Exchange and ■ ■ 2 Fat Exchanges can be served at lunch. This still leaves ■ 1 Fat Exchange for the sandwich and ■ 1 Fat Exchange as a garnish on the Perfection Salad.

Caution: There are two listings for mayonnaise. Two tablespoons low-calorie mayonnaise equal ■ 1 Fat Exchange (page 31) while 1 teaspoon regular mayonnaise equals ■ 1 Fat Exchange (page 29).

By saving ◣ ½ Milk Exchange from lunch, pudding can be enjoyed at dinner.

✳ EXCHANGE TIPS

For a hearty breakfast, ■ 1 Meat Exchange (1 egg) was added to the menu. If you enjoy drinking a glass of milk for breakfast, add ◣ ½ Milk Exchange from dinner to the breakfast menu.

Iceberg Ring filled with Tuna Salad is perfect for a ladies luncheon. Since ■ 1 Meat Exchange was transferred to breakfast, only ■ ■ 2 Meat Exchanges were left for lunch. A serving of Tuna Salad exactly fills this requirement.

A generous dinner is sure to follow this light lunch. At a barbecue, who can resist corn on the cob with plenty of butter? A perfect reward for saving ■ 1 Fat Exchange and ■ 1 Bread Exchange from your meal plan at lunch.

For an interesting relish plate, include celery and cucumber sticks, mushroom slices, green pepper rings, radish roses, summer squash slices along with carrot sticks and green onions. As the meal ends and snacks begin, serve your relish plate with a dip.

BREAKFAST

■ ■ 2 *Scrambled Eggs*

■ 1 *slice Toast with*
　　1 *teaspoon Butter*

■ 1 *slice Crisp Bacon*
■ ½ *Grapefruit*
■ 1 *cup Skim Milk*
■ *Coffee*

EXTRA EXCHANGES USED
■ 1 *Meat Exchange*
◣ ½ *Milk Exchange*

LUNCH

■ *Iceberg Ring* with*
■ ■ *Tuna Salad**
■ 5 *Saltines*
■ 2 *medium fresh or dietetic-pack Plums*
■ 1 *cup Skim Milk*

EXCHANGES NOT USED
■ 1 *Meat Exchange*
■ 1 *Fat Exchange*
■ 1 *Bread Exchange*

DINNER

■ ■ ■ *Ham Barbecue**
■ ■ *Potluck Potato Salad**

■ ■ 1 *ear Corn on the Cob with*
■ ■ 2 *teaspoons Butter*

Relish Plate:
■ 　*As Desired Vegetables*
◣ 　*carrot sticks*
◣ 　*green onions*

■ 1 *cup Watermelon*
■ *Coffee or Tea*

EXTRA EXCHANGES USED
■ 1 *Fat Exchange*
■ 1 *Bread Exchange*

EXCHANGES NOT USED
◣ ½ *Milk Exchange*

*see recipe section

Inviting appetizers

PICKLED MUSHROOMS

In small saucepan, combine ⅓ cup red wine vinegar, ⅓ cup water, 1 small onion, thinly sliced and separated in rings, 1 teaspoon salt, 2 teaspoons snipped parsley, 1 teaspoon prepared mustard, and non-caloric liquid sweetener equal to 1 tablespoon sugar. Bring to boiling. Add two 6-ounce cans mushroom crowns, drained; simmer 5 to 6 minutes. Pour into a bowl; cover. Chill several hours or overnight, stirring occasionally.

Drain; serve with cocktail picks. Makes 2 cups, an ■ As Desired Vegetable Exchange.

DOUBLE DECK COCKTAIL

2 cups chilled pineapple juice
2 cups chilled tomato juice

Into each glass, pour ⅓ cup pineapple juice; tip glass and slowly pour ⅓ cup tomato juice down side of glass. If desired, float thin lemon slices, halved, atop. Serves 6, each ■ 1 Fruit Exchange and an ■ As Desired Vegetable Exchange.

Double Deck Cocktail is trimmed with watercress. To fix drinks ahead of time, store in refrigerator; use within one hour.

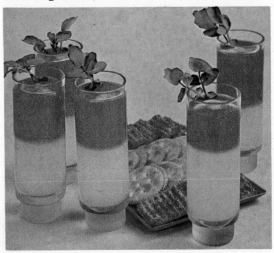

MARINATED ARTICHOKES

1 15-ounce can artichoke hearts
3 tablespoons lemon juice
Dash garlic salt
Non-caloric liquid sweetener equal to 2 teaspoons sugar
¼ teaspoon dried oregano, crushed
¼ teaspoon dried tarragon, crushed
Paprika

Drain artichokes, reserving liquid; cut artichokes into bite-size pieces. Combine artichokes, reserved liquid, and remaining ingredients; stir gently to blend. Cover; chill several hours. Sprinkle with paprika. Five artichokes equal ■ 1 Sturdy Vegetable Exchange.

TOMATO REFRESHER

2½ cups tomato juice
3 tablespoons lemon juice
⅛ teaspoon celery salt
1 teaspoon Worcestershire sauce
Non-caloric liquid sweetener equal to 1 teaspoon sugar
5 thin lemon slices

Combine first 5 ingredients; chill. Stir before serving. Float paper-thin lemon slices atop. Makes five 4-ounce servings. One serving equals an ■ As Desired Vegetable Exchange.

JAMAICAN SWIZZLE

¼ cup lime juice
3 dashes bitters
Non-caloric liquid sweetener equal to ¼ cup sugar
2 cups crushed ice
½ teaspoon rum flavoring

Put all ingredients in blender container; cover and blend at high speed for 10 to 15 seconds. Serve in cocktail glasses. Makes 3 servings, each a ■ Free Exchange.

PINEAPPLE PASSION

2 8½-ounce cans dietetic-pack
     pineapple tidbits
¼ cup lime juice
1 teaspoon rum flavoring

Combine all ingredients in blender container. Cover and run at high speed until pineapple is finely crushed. While blender is running, add 6 ice cubes, one at a time. Trim glasses with lime wedges. Serves 4, each ■ 1 Fruit Exchange.

SEAFOOD COCKTAIL SAUCE

¾ cup chili sauce
2 to 4 tablespoons lemon juice
1 tablespoon prepared horseradish
2 teaspoons Worcestershire sauce
½ teaspoon grated onion
    Few drops bottled hot pepper sauce

Combine all ingredients; salt to taste. Chill. Serve as a sauce for clams, shrimp, or oysters. Makes 1¼ cups, a ■ Free Exchange.

GAZPACHO

Combine one 10½-ounce can condensed beef broth, 2½ cups tomato juice, 3 tablespoons lemon juice, 2 tablespoons chopped onion, 1 clove garlic, sliced lengthwise, ¼ teaspoon bottled hot pepper sauce, ½ teaspoon salt, and dash freshly ground pepper. Cover; shake well. Chill 4 hours; remove garlic. Place mixture in freezer about 1 hour; *do not freeze.*

Meanwhile, chill 1 cup *each finely chopped* green pepper, cucumber, and tomato. Chill soup dishes. To serve, divide chilled vegetables among soup dishes. Pour soup over. Serves 8 to 10, each an ■ As Desired Vegetable Exchange.

BEEF-O-MATO SOUP

Combine one 10½-ounce can condensed beef broth, 2 cups tomato juice, ½ teaspoon instant minced onion, 1 teaspoon Worcestershire sauce, and 1 tablespoon lemon juice; chill. Makes 3½ cups, a ■ Free Exchange.

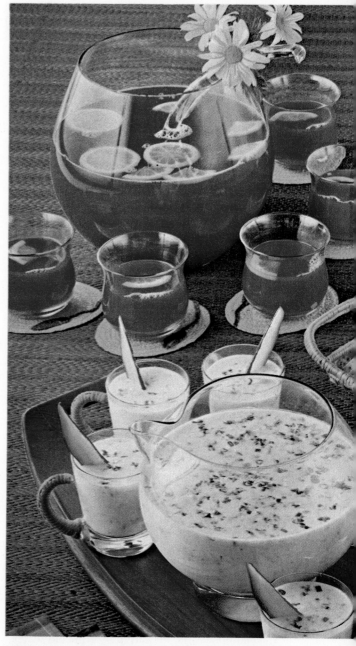

Glistening **Beef-O-Mato Soup is topped with paper thin lemon floaters. It's a breeze to make; simply combine and chill. The creamy appetizer sporting cuke sticks is** *Cuke-Buttermilk Soup:* **Pare 2 cucumbers; remove seeds and grate. Add 1 quart buttermilk, 1 tablespoon chopped green onion, ¼ cup snipped parsley, 1 teaspoon salt, and dash pepper. Cover and chill. Serves 4, each ■ 1 Milk Exchange.**

Salads and vegetables

MOLDED CRANBERRY WALDORFS

- 1 1-pint bottle (2 cups) low-calorie cranberry-juice cocktail
- 1 4-serving envelope low-calorie strawberry-flavored gelatin
- ¼ teaspoon salt
- 1 cup chopped, unpared apple
- ½ cup chopped celery

Bring *1 cup* of the cranberry-juice cocktail to boiling; stir in gelatin till dissolved. Add remaining cranberry-juice and salt. Chill till partially set. Stir in apple and celery. Pour into 1-quart mold. Chill till set. Unmold on crisp greens. Makes 4 servings, each ½ Fruit Exchange.

LIME-APPLESAUCE MOLD

- 1 1-pound can dietetic-pack applesauce
- 1 4-serving envelope low-calorie lime-flavored gelatin
- 1 cup low-calorie lemon-lime carbonated beverage

Combine applesauce and gelatin in saucepan. Cook and stir till gelatin dissolves. Slowly stir in carbonated beverage. Pour into individual molds or 3-cup mold. Chill till firm. Makes 4 servings, each 1 Fruit Exchange.

PERFECTION SALAD

In saucepan, soften 2 envelopes (2 tablespoons) unflavored gelatin in ½ cup cold water. Add non-caloric liquid sweetener equal to ½ cup sugar, ½ teaspoon salt, and 1 cup water; stir over low heat to dissolve gelatin. Add 2 cups water, ½ cup vinegar, and 2 tablespoons lemon juice. Chill till mixture is partially set.

Stir in 2 cups finely shredded cabbage, 1 cup chopped celery, and ¼ cup *each* chopped green pepper and canned pimiento. Pour into 8½x4½ x2½-inch loaf dish. Chill till firm. Each serving equals As Desired Vegetable Exchange.

CABBAGE PINEAPPLE SLAW

Combine 3 cups shredded crisp cabbage, one 8-ounce can (1 cup) dietetic-pack pineapple tidbits, drained, 1 cup diced apple, ½ cup chopped celery, and ¼ cup light raisins. Toss with ½ cup low-calorie mayonnaise until well coated. Serve in lettuce-lined bowl. Garnish with apple wedges. Makes 6 servings, each 1 Fruit Exchange and ½ Fat Exchange.

BLENDER CUCUMBER SALAD

- 1 large cucumber, pared
- 1 4-serving envelope low-calorie lemon-flavored gelatin

Slice cucumber into blender container. Cover; blend on high speed till pureed. Stop blender to push cucumber down from side of container. Add water to puree, if necessary, to make 1 cup. Dissolve gelatin in 1¼ cups boiling water; add cucumber. Chill till partially thickened; stir occasionally. Pour into 3-cup mold. Chill till set. Serves 4, each As Desired Vegetable Exchange. Serve with Cottage Cheese Dressing.

COTTAGE CHEESE DRESSING

- 1 cup cottage cheese, not creamed
- Non-caloric liquid sweetener equal to 2 tablespoons sugar
- 4 teaspoons lemon juice
- ½ cup skim milk

Combine cottage cheese, sweetener, and lemon juice in blender container; blend till creamy. Add milk, a tablespoon at a time, till of desired consistency. Makes 1 cup. Two tablespoons equal ½ Meat Exchange.

Cool summer salads

Iceberg Ring with crisp lettuce in lime-fla- → vored gelatin proudly displays a peak of Tuna Salad—a refreshing combination.

ICEBERG RING

■

Fill the center with your favorite meat salad—

Dissolve two 4-serving envelopes low-calorie lime-flavored gelatin and ½ teaspoon salt in 2 cups boiling water. Stir in 1½ cups cold water and 2 tablespoons vinegar. Chill till mixture is slightly thickened.

Fold in 3 cups coarsely chopped Iceberg lettuce and ¼ cup thinly sliced green onion. Pour into 5-cup ring mold. Chill till firm, about 3 hours. Makes 6 to 8 servings. Each serving equals ■ As Desired Vegetable Exchange. If desired, fill center with Tuna Salad.

TUNA SALAD

■ ■ □

- ½ cup low-calorie mayonnaise
- 1 tablespoon lemon juice
- 2 tablespoons capers
- ¼ teaspoon salt
  Dash pepper
- 2 6½-ounce cans chilled dietetic-pack tuna, drained and broken in pieces
- ¾ cup diced cucumber

Combine first 5 ingredients for dressing. Combine tuna and cucumber. Just before serving, toss tuna with dressing. Serves 6, each ■ ■ 2 Meat Exchanges, □ 1 Fat Exchange.

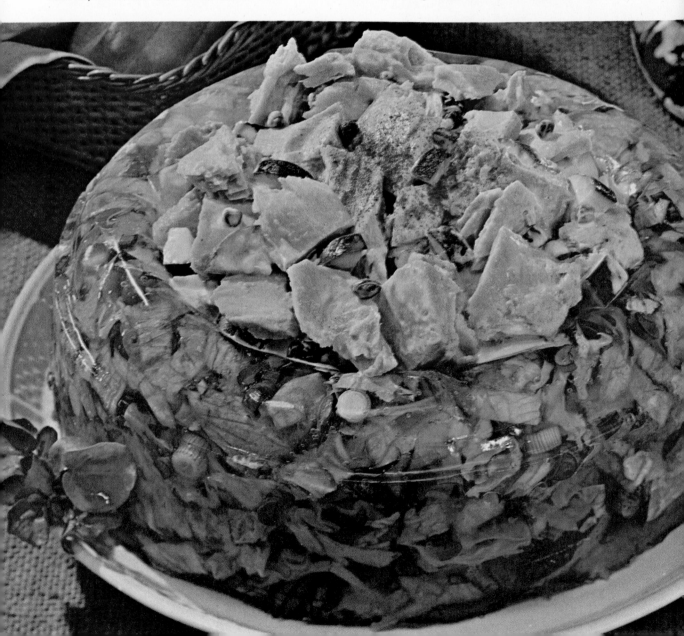

GOURMET DRESSING

■

1¼ teaspoons unflavored gelatin
1½ cups tomato juice
2½ teaspoons dry salad dressing mix
2 tablespoons vinegar

Soften gelatin in ½ *cup* tomato juice; bring to a boil stirring to dissolve gelatin. Add salad dressing mix, vinegar, and remaining tomato juice. Blend thoroughly; chill. Stir before serving. Makes 1⅔ cups, a ■ Free Exchange.

TOMATO DRESSING

■

Combine one 8-ounce can tomato sauce, 2 tablespoons tarragon vinegar, 1 teaspoon onion juice, 1 teaspoon Worcestershire sauce, ½ teaspoon salt, ½ teaspoon dillweed, and ½ teaspoon dried basil, crushed. Cover and shake well; chill. Shake before serving. Makes 1 cup. Two tablespoons equals ■ 1 Fat Exchange.

SLIM-TRIM DRESSING

■

Keep this tangy dressing on hand for tossed salads—

1 tablespoon cornstarch
½ teaspoon dry mustard
1 cup cold water

. . .

¼ cup vinegar
¼ cup catsup
½ teaspoon paprika
½ teaspoon prepared horseradish
½ teaspoon Worcestershire sauce
Dash non-caloric liquid sweetener
Dash salt
1 clove garlic, halved

Combine cornstarch and mustard in small saucepan. Gradually stir in water. Cook over medium heat, stirring constantly, till mixture thickens; cool. Add remaining ingredients except garlic. Beat till smooth. Add garlic; cover; store in refrigerator. Shake well before using. Makes 1⅓ cups. Up to 2 tablespoons a ■ Free Exchange.

VEGETABLE SEASONING GUIDE

Artichokes: bay leaves, thyme
Asparagus: caraway seed, mustard, sesame seed, tarragon
Green beans: basil, bay leaves, curry, dill, marjoram, mustard, oregano, savory, sesame seed, tarragon, thyme
Lima beans: celery seed, chili powder, curry, oregano, sage
Baked beans: cloves, ginger, oregano
Beets: allspice, bay leaves, caraway seed, celery seed, cloves, ginger, nutmeg, savory, tarragon, thyme
Broccoli: caraway seed, mustard, oregano
Brussels sprouts: caraway seed, mustard, nutmeg, sage
Cabbage: allspice, basil, caraway seed, celery seed, dill, mustard, nutmeg, oregano, savory, tarragon
Carrots: allspice, bay leaves, caraway seed, celery seed, chives, curry, dill, ginger, mace, marjoram, mint, nutmeg, savory, tarragon, thyme
Cauliflower: caraway seed, celery seed, curry, dill, mustard, nutmeg, oregano, savory, tarragon
Corn: celery seed, chili powder, chives

Eggplant: allspice, basil, bay leaves, chili powder, marjoram, sage, thyme
Mushrooms: rosemary, tarragon, thyme
Onions: basil, bay leaves, caraway seed, chili powder, curry, ginger, mustard, nutmeg, oregano, sage, thyme
Peas: basil, chili powder, dill, marjoram, mint, mustard, oregano, rosemary, sage
Potatoes, sweet: allspice, cardamom, cinnamon, cloves, ginger, nutmeg
Potatoes, white: basil, bay leaves, caraway seed, celery seed, chives, dill, mace, mustard, oregano, rosemary, savory, sesame seed, thyme
Spinach: allspice, basil, cinnamon, dill, mace, marjoram, nutmeg, oregano, rosemary, sesame seed
Squash, summer: basil, bay leaves, mace, marjoram, mustard, rosemary
Squash, winter: allspice, basil, cinnamon, cloves, ginger, nutmeg
Tomatoes: basil, bay leaves, caraway seed, celery seed, curry, dill, oregano, rosemary, sage, sesame seed, thyme
Turnips: allspice, caraway seed, celery seed, dill, oregano

BEAN-STUFFED TOMATOES

■

Cook one 9-ounce package frozen Italian green beans using package directions. Drain thoroughly. Place in bowl with one 3-ounce can sliced mushrooms, drained, ⅓ cup low-calorie Italian salad dressing, ¼ cup sliced green onion, ¼ teaspoon salt, and dash pepper; toss. Refrigerate 2 hours, tossing occasionally.

Meanwhile, cut thin slice from tops of 6 medium tomatoes. Scoop out center, leaving shell about ¼-inch thick. Invert on paper towels to drain; chill. At serving time season shells with salt and fill with bean mixture. Serves 6, each ■ As Desired Vegetable Exchange.

BROILED TOMATOES

■

    3 medium-size tomatoes
      Salt and pepper
  ¼ teaspoon dried oregano *or*
      basil, crushed
    2 tablespoons low-calorie Italian
      or French salad dressing

Core tomatoes and cut in half crosswise. Make shallow crisscross cuts on surface of tomatoes. Season cut surfaces with salt and pepper. Sprinkle with oregano or basil; drizzle with salad dressing. Broil, cut side up, 3 inches from heat about 5 minutes or till heated through. Serves 6, each ■ As Desired Vegetable Exchange.

POTLUCK POTATO SALAD

■ ■

Cook 5 medium potatoes in jackets; peel and cube. Pour ¼ cup low-calorie French salad dressing over warm potatoes; chill 2 hours. Add 1 cup chopped celery, ⅓ cup chopped onion, 4 hard-cooked eggs, sliced, and 1 teaspoon salt. Combine ½ cup low-calorie mayonnaise and 2 teaspoons prepared mustard; carefully mix with potato mixture. Add 1 teaspoon celery seed, if desired. Chill 4 hours. Makes 8 servings, each ■ 1 Bread Exchange and ■ 1 Fat Exchange.

Perfect partner for steak

Juicy red tomatoes filled to the brim with →
marinated green beans and mushrooms
make Bean-stuffed Tomatoes a big bonus.

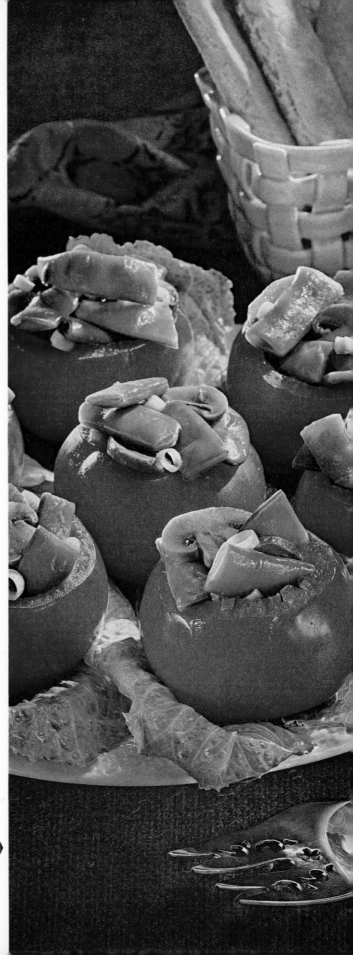

58

Hearty main dishes

MAIN DISH SEASONING GUIDE

Beef: allspice, basil, bay leaves, caraway seed, celery seed, chili powder, cumin, ginger, mace, marjoram, oregano, rosemary, savory, tarragon, thyme
Veal: bay leaves, ginger, mace, marjoram, mint, oregano, rosemary, savory, thyme
Pork: bay leaves, caraway seed, chili powder, cloves, curry, marjoram, oregano, rosemary, sage, thyme
Ham: allspice, cloves, ginger, mustard
Lamb: allspice, basil, bay leaves, curry, dill, ginger, marjoram, mint, oregano, rosemary, savory, thyme

Poultry: bay leaves, curry, ginger, marjoram, oregano, rosemary, sage, saffron, savory, tarragon, thyme
Fish: allspice, bay leaves, celery seed, curry, marjoram, mustard, oregano, sage, savory, tarragon, thyme
Shellfish: basil, bay leaves, chili powder, curry, marjoram
Eggs: basil, celery seed, chili powder, cumin, curry, marjoram, mustard, rosemary, savory, tarragon, thyme
Cheese: caraway seed, cumin, ginger, mace, mustard, oregano, rosemary, sage

CURRIED CHICKEN BREASTS
■ ■

Skin, bone, and halve lengthwise 3 broiler-fryer chicken breasts (2 pounds). Sprinkle with ½ teaspoon seasoned salt and dash paprika; place in 11x7x1½-inch baking pan. In a small saucepan, drain the liquid from one 3-ounce can broiled sliced mushrooms; add 1 chicken bouillon cube. Heat and stir till bouillon is dissolved.

To the mushroom liquid add sliced mushrooms, ¼ cup sauterne, ½ teaspoon instant minced onion, ¼ teaspoon curry powder, and dash pepper; pour over chicken. Cover with foil and bake at 350° for 40 minutes. Uncover and bake 20 minutes longer. Serve with pan juices. Makes 6 servings each ■ ■ 2 Meat Exchanges.

BREAD STUFFING
■

In small saucepan, dissolve 1 chicken bouillon cube in ½ to ¾ cup boiling water. Add ¼ cup chopped onion and simmer 5 minutes. Meanwhile, combine 4 cups ½-inch dry bread cubes (6 slices), ½ teaspoon poultry seasoning, ½ teaspoon dried sage, crushed, ¼ teaspoon salt, and ⅛ teaspoon pepper. Pour onion-broth mixture over bread, tossing gently to moisten. Makes enough stuffing for 4 to 5 pound chicken (double recipe for 10 pound turkey). Each ⅓ cup serving equals ■ 1 Bread Exchange.

FRENCH HERBED CHICKEN
■ ■ ■ ■

- 1 3-pound ready-to-cook broiler-fryer chicken, cut up
- 1 tablespoon shortening
- 1 8-ounce can (1 cup) small whole onions, drained
- ½ cup coarsely chopped carrot
- 1 clove garlic, crushed
- 2 tablespoons snipped parsley
- ¼ teaspoon dried thyme, crushed
- 1 2-ounce can sliced mushrooms
- 1 cup sauterne
- 2 or 3 branches celery, cut up
- 1 medium bay leaf

In skillet, brown chicken in hot fat. Season with salt and pepper and place in 2-quart casserole. Drain excess fat in skillet; add remaining ingredients except celery and bay leaf. Heat, scraping up browned pieces. Pour over chicken. Tuck in celery and bay leaf. Cover and bake at 350° for 1¼ hours. Remove bay leaf and celery. Serves 4 each ■ ■ ■ ■ 4 Meat Exchanges and ■ 1 Sturdy Vegetable Exchange.

Perfect for company

French Herbed Chicken is easy to prepare →but elegant to eat. The subtle blend of seasonings is sure to delight your friends.

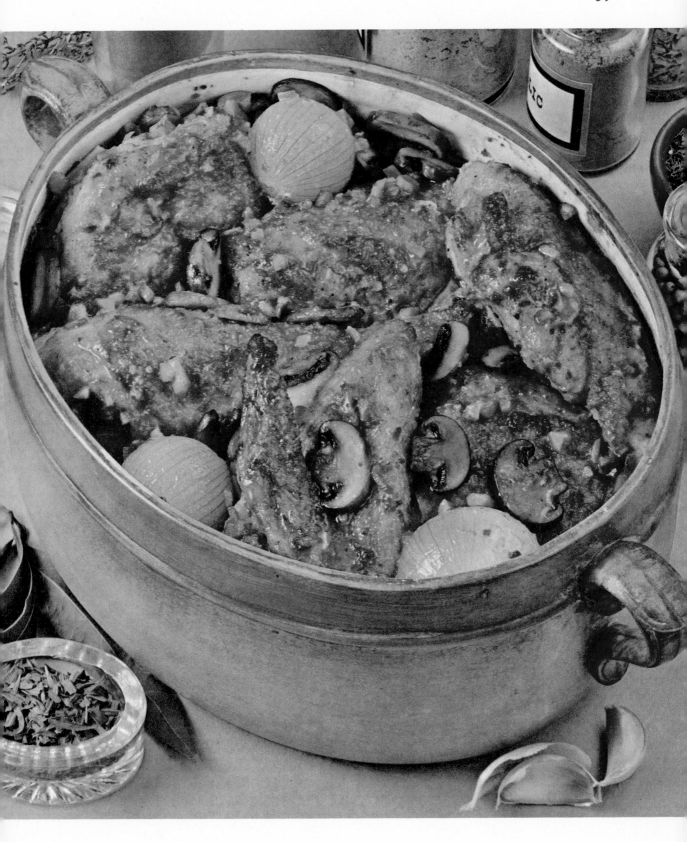

BARBECUED PORK AND BEANS
■ ■ ■

Combine one 1-pound can baked beans in tomato sauce (no pork) and 2 tablespoons chopped onion; place in 10x6x1½-inch baking dish. Trim fat off four 5-ounce lean rib pork chops; season. Spread generously with prepared mustard and catsup; sprinkle with lemon juice and non-caloric liquid sweetener. Place over beans.

Bake at 325° for 1¼ hours. Top each chop with 1 onion slice and 1 lemon slice; secure with wooden pick. Bake 15 minutes more. Serves 4, each ■ ■ ■ 3 Meat Exchanges and ■ 1 Bread Exchange (¼ cup beans per serving).

HAM BARBECUE
■ ■ ■

½ cup catsup
2 tablespoons finely chopped onion
1 tablespoon Worcestershire sauce
2 teaspoons lemon juice
2 teaspoons prepared mustard
¼ teaspoon chili powder
   Non-caloric liquid sweetener equal to 1 tablespoon sugar
1 fully cooked ham slice (1½ pounds)

Combine first 7 ingredients for sauce. Slash fat edge of ham at 2-inch intervals. Brush meat liberally with sauce and let stand 1 hour. Broil 3 to 4 inches from heat 5 to 6 minutes per side, turning once and brushing with sauce. Serves 8, each ■ ■ ■ 3 Meat Exchanges.

SKILLET SPAGHETTI
■ ■ ◣ ■ ■

In large skillet, break up 1 pound ground beef. Add one 6-ounce can tomato paste, one 1-pint 2-ounce can tomato juice, 3 cups water, 1½ to 2 teaspoons chili powder, 1 teaspoon garlic salt, 1 teaspoon salt, 1 teaspoon sugar, 1 teaspoon dried oregano, crushed, and 2 tablespoons instant minced onion. Cover; bring to boil; simmer 30 minutes; stir occasionally.

Add one 7-ounce package spaghetti; stir to separate strands. Cover; simmer 30 minutes or till spaghetti is tender. Stir frequently. Serves 4 to 6. Each cup equals ■ ■ ◣ 2½ Meat Exchanges, ■ 1 Bread Exchange, and ■ 1 Sturdy Vegetable Exchange. Three tablespoons Parmesan cheese equals ◣ ½ Meat Exchange.

FAVORITE BEEF LOAF
■ ■ ■ ■

1½ pounds ground beef
⅓ cup cracker crumbs
2 beaten eggs
½ cup tomato juice
¼ cup finely chopped onion
2 tablespoons chopped green pepper
1¼ teaspoons salt
   Dash dried thyme, crushed
   Dash dried marjoram, crushed

Combine all ingredients; mix well. Shape in a loaf in shallow baking dish. Bake at 350° for 1¼ hours. Serves 8, each ■ ■ ■ 3 Meat Exchanges and ■ 1 Sturdy Vegetable Exchange.

INDIVIDUAL POT ROASTS
■ ■ ■ ■ ■ ■

In Dutch oven brown four 6-ounce pieces boneless beef chuck slowly in 1 tablespoon cooking oil. Season with 1 teaspoon salt and dash pepper. Add 1 cup water. Cover; simmer for 1 hour; add water if necessary. Add 4 pared and halved carrots, 3 quartered medium onions, and 4 quartered medium potatoes to meat. Simmer 45 minutes or till tender. Serve with skimmed juice. Serves 4, each ■ ■ ■ ■ 4 Meat Exchanges, ■ 1 Sturdy Vegetable Exchange, ■ 1 Bread Exchange, and ■ 1 Fat Exchange.

CORNED-BEEF DINNER
■ ■ ■ ■ ■ ■

1 3-pound corned-beef brisket
1 onion, chopped
2 garlic cloves, minced
2 bay leaves
6 small potatoes, pared
6 small carrots, pared
6 cabbage wedges (1 medium head)

Place corned beef in Dutch oven; barely cover with hot water. Add onion, garlic, and bay leaves. Cover; *simmer* about 3 hours or till tender. Remove meat from liquid; add potatoes and carrots. Cover; bring to boil; cook 10 minutes. Add cabbage; cook 20 minutes. Carve meat across the grain, making thin slices. Serves 6, each ■ ■ ■ ■ 4 Meat Exchanges, ■ 1 Sturdy Vegetable Exchange, ■ As Desired Vegetable Exchange, and ■ 1 Bread Exchange.

DEVILED SWISS STEAK
■ ■ ■

  1 3-pound beef round steak
1½ teaspoons salt
1½ teaspoons dry mustard
  ¼ teaspoon pepper
  2 tablespoons cooking oil
  1 6-ounce can mushrooms
  1 tablespoon Worcestershire sauce

Trim fat from meat. Combine salt, dry mustard, and pepper. Sprinkle over meat and pound with mallet. In heavy skillet, brown steak slowly on both sides in hot oil. Drain off excess fat. Drain mushrooms, reserving ½ cup liquid. Add mushroom liquid and Worcestershire to skillet. Cover tightly and cook over very low heat for 1¾ to 2 hours or till tender. Last few minutes, add mushrooms and heat through. Skim fat from sauce before serving. Makes 8 servings, each ■ ■ ■ 3 Meat Exchanges.

PAMPERED BEEF FILLETS
■ ■ ■

  1 3-ounce can chopped mushrooms, drained (½ cup)
  ¼ cup snipped green onion
  1 cup Burgundy
  1 teaspoon salt
  9 4-ounce beef fillets (1 inch thick)
  9 fresh mushroom crowns (optional)

In saucepan, combine chopped mushrooms, onion, and ½ cup water; simmer 5 minutes. Stir in Burgundy, salt, and dash pepper. Place fillets in plastic bag; pour in wine sauce; fasten bag securely. Marinate in refrigerator several hours. Remove fillets, reserving sauce. Broil 3 inches from heat 7 minutes; turn and broil 6 minutes. Top with mushroom crowns (X-shape slash in top) last few minutes of broiling. Sprinkle with snipped parsley. Heat sauce and serve. Each fillet equals ■ ■ ■ 3 Meat Exchanges.

Juicy and tender, Deviled Swiss Steak is cooked slowly in a small amount of liquid spiced with Worcestershire sauce and dry mustard. Garnish with mushroom crowns.

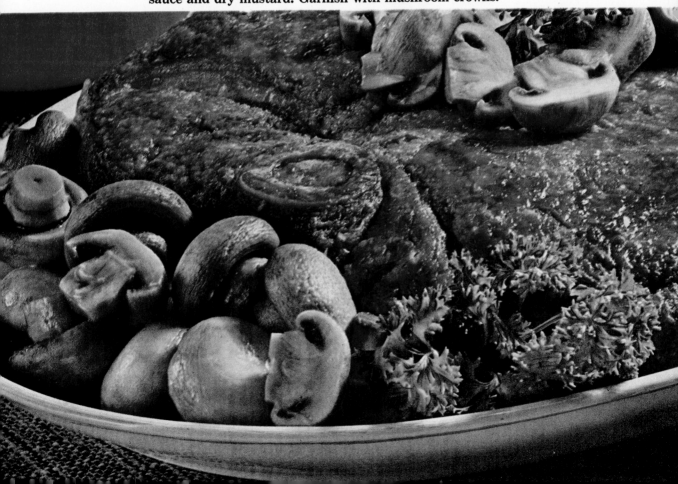

LAMB CHOPS ORIENTAL

■ ■ ■

    6 4-ounce lamb shoulder chops,
      ½-inch thick
    ½ cup soy sauce
    ½ cup water
    1 clove garlic, minced

Score fat edges of chops. Place in shallow baking dish. Combine soy sauce, water, and garlic; pour over chops. Cover. Let stand in refrigerator several hours or overnight. Arrange marinated chops on broiler pan rack. Broil 3 inches from heat about 10 minutes. Turn chops and broil 5 to 8 minutes longer. Makes 6 servings, each ■ ■ ■ 3 Meat Exchanges.

SMOKED SALMON BAKE

■ ■ ■

Place 1 pound of salmon steaks *or* other fish steaks in greased 10x6x1½-inch baking dish. Sprinkle with ½ teaspoon salt and dash pepper. Combine one 3-ounce can chopped mushrooms, drained, ¼ cup catsup, 2 tablespoons snipped green onions, 2 tablespoons lemon juice, and 10 drops liquid smoke. Spoon over fish.

Bake in moderate oven (350°) for 25 to 30 minutes or until fish flakes with a fork. Makes 5 servings each ■ ■ ■ 3 Meat Exchanges.

FLOUNDER IN WINE

■ ■ ■

Easy to prepare, elegant to eat—

    1 pound flounder fillets or
      other fish fillets
    ½ teaspoon salt
      Dash pepper
    2 tomatoes, peeled and sliced
    ¼ cup dry white wine
    ½ teaspoon dried basil, crushed
    ½ cup shredded sharp process
      American cheese

Place fillets in greased 11x7x1½-inch baking pan. Sprinkle with ½ teaspoon salt and pepper. Arrange tomatoes on top; sprinkle with salt. Carefully pour wine over all; sprinkle with basil. Bake in moderate oven (350°) for 20 minutes. Sprinkle with cheese and bake 5 to 10 minutes or until fish flakes with fork. Makes 5 servings each ■ ■ ■ 3 Meat Exchanges.

POACHED SALMON

■ ■ ■

    6 7-ounce frozen salmon steaks
    1 quart water
    1½ tablespoons salt
    2 tablespoons lemon juice

Thaw frozen salmon. In a skillet, bring water to boiling. Add salt and lemon juice. Lower salmon steaks into water. Simmer 8 to 10 minutes. Remove fish from liquid with slotted spoon. Chill or serve hot. Serve with Cucumber-dill Sauce and lemon wedges. *Half* of one salmon steak equals ■ ■ ■ 3 Meat Exchanges.

CUCUMBER-DILL SAUCE

▶

    1 medium cucumber
    ½ cup plain yogurt
    ¼ cup low-calorie mayonnaise
    1 tablespoon snipped parsley
    2 teaspoons lemon juice
    2 teaspoons grated onion
    ½ teaspoon dried dillweed
    ¼ teaspoon salt
      Dash pepper

Shred cucumber to make 1 cup; combine with remaining ingredients. Blend well; chill. Serve on Poached Salmon or other fish. Garnish with cucumber twist. Makes 1½ cups. Three tablespoons equals ▶ ½ Fat Exchange.

TARTARE SAUCE

▶

    ½ cup low-calorie mayonnaise
    1 tablespoon finely chopped dill pickle
    1 teaspoon finely chopped onion
    1 teaspoon snipped parsley
    1 teaspoon finely chopped canned
      pimiento

Combine all ingredients. Chill thoroughly. Serve with fish. Makes about ½ cup of sauce. Each tablespoon equals ▶ ½ Fat Exchange.

A treat for any season

**Poached Salmon and Cucumber-dill Sauce →
is perfect any season of the year. Garnish
with juicy lemon wedges, cherry tomatoes.**

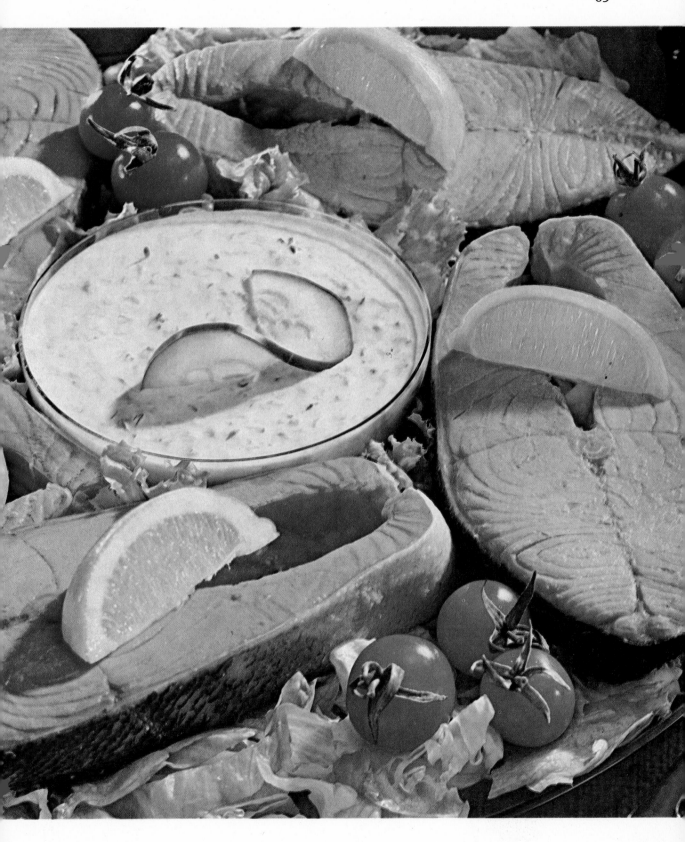

Casual suppers

WELSH RAREBIT
■ ■ ◣ ■

2 cups shredded sharp process cheese
¾ cup skim milk
1 teaspoon dry mustard
1 teaspoon Worcestershire sauce
Dash cayenne
1 well-beaten egg

Heat cheese and milk over low heat, stirring constantly till cheese melts. Add seasonings. Stir a small amount of hot mixture into egg; return to hot mixture. Cook and stir over low heat till thickened and creamy. Serve immediately over 4 slices toast. Serves 4, each ■ ■ ◣ 2½ Meat Exchanges and ■ 1 Bread Exchange.

MACARONI AND CHEESE
■ ■

Cook 1½ cups elbow macaroni using package directions; drain. Simmer ¼ cup chopped onion in ¼ cup water, covered, 5 minutes; add ¾ cup skim milk and 1½ cups shredded sharp process American cheese. Cook and stir till cheese melts; pour over macaroni. Add 2 tablespoons chopped canned pimiento; mix well. Turn into 1½-quart casserole; bake covered at 350° for 35 minutes. Dash with paprika. Serves 6, each ■ 1 Meat Exchange and ■ 1 Bread Exchange.

FRANK-VEGETABLE MEDLEY
■ ■ ■ ■

5 frankfurters, cut in 1-inch pieces
½ cup long-grain rice
1 8-ounce can (1 cup) tomato sauce
1 10-ounce package frozen mixed
   vegetables, slightly thawed
¼ cup chopped onion
   Dash bottled hot pepper sauce

In 2-quart casserole, combine all ingredients; break up vegetables. Stir in 1 cup water and 1 teaspoon salt. Bake, covered, at 375° for 1 hour; stir occasionally. Serves 5, each ■ 1 Meat Exchange, ■ 1 Bread Exchange, ■ 1 Fat Exchange, and ■ 1 Sturdy Vegetable Exchange.

SLIM-JIM TUNA SALAD
■ ■ ■

Combine ¾ cup wine vinegar, non-caloric liquid sweetener equal to 2 teaspoons sugar, 1½ teaspoons dried basil, crushed, ¼ teaspoon salt, and dash pepper; chill. Break up two 6½-ounce cans dietetic-pack tuna, drained.

Add 8 cups torn lettuce, 1½ cups cherry tomatoes, halved, ½ medium onion, thinly sliced and separated in rings, 1 medium cucumber, sliced, and ½ cup sliced celery. Add dressing; toss lightly. Serves 7, each ■ ■ 2 Meat Exchanges and ■ As Desired Vegetable Exchange.

CHEF'S SALAD
■ ■ ■ ■

5 cups mixed salad greens
4 1-ounce slices *each* Swiss cheese
   and boiled ham, cut in
   julienne strips
8 cherry tomatoes
4 hard-cooked eggs, quartered
¼ cup finely snipped green onion
½ cup low-calorie salad dressing

Tear greens in bite-size pieces into 4 salad bowls. Layer atop each bowl: ¼ of the ham and cheese strips, 2 cherry tomatoes, halved, 4 egg quarters, and 1 tablespoon green onion. Drizzle with 2 tablespoons dressing; serve immediately. Serves 4, each ■ ■ ■ 3 Meat Exchanges and ■ As Desired Vegetable Exchange.

CHILI CON CARNE
■ ■ ■ ■ ■ ■

Cook 1 pound lean ground beef, 1 cup chopped onion, and ¾ cup chopped green pepper till meat is lightly browned and vegetables are tender. Spoon off fat. Stir in one 1-pound can tomatoes, broken up, one 1-pound can dark red kidney beans, drained, one 8-ounce can tomato sauce, 1 teaspoon salt, 1 to 2 teaspoons chili powder, and 1 bay leaf. Cover and simmer for 1 hour. Remove bay leaf. Serves 4, each ■ ■ ■ ■ 4 Meat Exchanges, ■ ■ 2 Bread Exchanges, and ■ 1 Fat Exchange.

NO CRUST PIZZA
■ ■ ■

Drain one 3-ounce can chopped mushrooms, adding water if necessary to equal ⅓ cup liquid. Combine liquid, 1 cup soft bread crumbs, 1 slightly beaten egg, ½ teaspoon salt, and dash pepper; let stand 5 minutes. Add 1 pound ground chuck, ½ teaspoon dried oregano, crushed, and *half* the mushrooms; mix lightly.

In a 9-inch pie plate form a "meat" crust. Cut 2 slices mozzarella cheese into 8 triangles; layer 4 over meat. Top with one 5½-ounce can pizza sauce, ¼ cup chopped onion, 2 tablespoons chopped green pepper, and remaining mushrooms. Dash with oregano. Bake at 350° for 55 minutes. Top with remaining cheese; bake 5 minutes. Let stand 10 minutes before serving. Serves 8, each ■ ■ ■ 3 Meat Exchanges.

SKILLETBURGERS
■ ■ ■ ■ ■

Cook 1 pound ground beef and 1 cup *each* chopped onion and celery till meat is browned. Drain off fat. Stir in two 8-ounce cans tomato sauce, ½ cup water, dash hot pepper sauce, ¾ teaspoon salt, ½ teaspoon monosodium glutamate, and ¼ teaspoon chili powder. Simmer uncovered 30 minutes.

Serve on ½ bun. Serves 8, each ■ ■ 2 Meat Exchanges, ■ 1 Bread Exchange, ■ 1 Sturdy Vegetable Exchange, ■ 1 Fat Exchange.

DEVILED BEEF PATTIES
■ ■ ■ ■

Combine 1 pound ground beef, 1 egg, ¼ cup chili sauce, 1 teaspoon prepared mustard, 1 teaspoon prepared horseradish, 1 teaspoon instant minced onion, 1 teaspoon Worcestershire sauce, ½ teaspoon salt, and dash pepper. Mix well. Shape into 4 patties.

Broil 3 inches from heat for 5 minutes; turn and broil 4 minutes longer or till done. Serve on plain toasted ½ hamburger bun. Makes 4 servings, each ■ ■ ■ 3 Meat Exchanges and ■ 1 Bread Exchange.

Perfect for the grill

Having company over for a cookout? Serve →
Deviled Beef Patties on an open-faced bun.
Top with cherry tomatoes and onion rings.

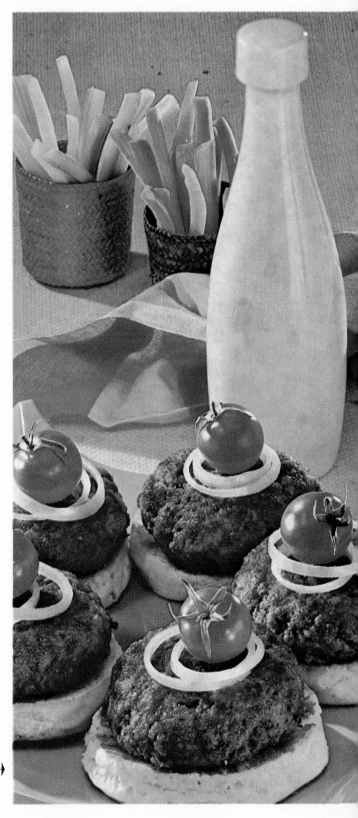

66

TUNA SALAD SANDWICH

■ ■ ■ ■ ■

Drain one 6½-ounce can dietetic-pack tuna; break tuna in chunks and sprinkle with 1 tablespoon lemon juice. Combine tuna, 2 hard-cooked eggs, coarsely chopped, ⅓ cup low-calorie mayonnaise, ¼ cup thinly sliced dill pickle, 2 tablespoons snipped green onion, ¼ teaspoon salt, and dash pepper. Mix gently and chill.

Split and toast 2 English muffins. Spread *each* muffin half with 1 teaspoon low-calorie mayonnaise; layer with Boston or Bibb lettuce and 3 thin tomato slices atop. Season lightly with salt. Pile tuna salad mixture on top. Makes 4 sandwiches. Each sandwich equals ■ ■ 2 Meat Exchanges, ■ 1 Bread Exchange, ■ As Desired Vegetable Exchange, and ■ 1 Fat Exchange.

CORNED BEEF SLAWICH

■ ■ ■ ■ ■

    ⅔ cup low-calorie mayonnaise
    2 teaspoons prepared mustard
    4 cups finely shredded cabbage
    ¼ cup snipped green onion
    6 slices whole wheat bread, toasted
    1 12-ounce can corned beef, chilled and sliced in 12 slices

Blend mayonnaise and mustard. Combine cabbage and green onion; add mayonnaise mixture and toss to coat. Spoon coleslaw onto toast slices and arrange 2 slices corned beef on top of each. Garnish with cherry tomatoes. Makes 6 servings, each ■ ■ 2 Meat Exchanges, ■ 1 Bread Exchange, ■ As Desired Vegetable Exchange, and ■ 1 Fat Exchange.

PEACHY HAM SWISSER

■ ■ ■ ■ ■ ■ ■

Toast 4 slices rye bread; spread each slice with 1 teaspoon low-calorie mayonnaise. Layer *each* with lettuce, 2 slices boiled ham, 1 slice process Swiss cheese, and 2 dietetic-pack peach halves.

Combine ½ cup low-calorie mayonnaise, 2 tablespoons skim milk, 2 tablespoons chili sauce, and 1 tablespoon finely chopped dill pickle. Drizzle about 3 tablespoons over each sandwich. Makes 4 sandwiches, each ■ ■ ■ 3 Meat Exchanges, ■ 1 Bread Exchange, ■ 1 Fruit Exchange, ■ 1 Fat Exchange, and ■ As Desired Vegetable Exchange.

TURKEY-CHEESE SANDWICH

■ ■ ■ ■ ■◤

    1 10-ounce package frozen asparagus spears
    2 tablespoons finely chopped onion
    ½ cup low-calorie Italian salad dressing
    ¼ teaspoon freshly ground pepper
    3 tablespoons low-calorie mayonnaise
    4 slices white bread, toasted
    8 1-ounce slices cooked turkey
    4 slices (4 ounces) process Swiss cheese, halved diagonally

Cook asparagus spears according to package directions; drain well. Combine onion, salad dressing, and pepper; pour over asparagus in saucepan. Bring to boil.

Spread mayonnaise on toast. Top *each* with 2 slices of turkey, several hot asparagus spears, and 2 triangles of cheese. Broil 5 inches from heat for 2 to 3 minutes, just till cheese melts. Makes 4 servings, each ■ ■ ■ 3 Meat Exchanges, ■ 1 Bread Exchange, ■ As Desired Vegetable Exchange, and ◤ ½ Fat Exchange.

SALAD SUPPER SANDWICH

■ ■ ■ ■ ■ ■

    4 slices rye bread, toasted
    4 teaspoons softened butter Romaine
    2 1-ounce slices sharp process American cheese, cut in julienne strips
    4 slices pressed ham
    4 slices Cotto salami
    1 large tomato, cut in 8 slices
    2 hard-cooked eggs, sliced
    4 tablespoons low-calorie French salad dressing

Spread each slice of toast with 1 teaspoon butter. For *each* sandwich, layer in order: Romaine, cheese, ham, salami, tomato, and egg; drizzle with 1 tablespoon French dressing. Serves 4, each ■ ■ ■ 3 Meat Exchanges, ■ 1 Bread Exchange, ■ 1 Fat Exchange, and ■ As Desired Vegetable Exchange.

Tasty meal-sized sandwich

For a luncheon treat serve Turkey-cheese → Sandwich. Coupled with a fruit dessert and beverage, your noon meal is complete.

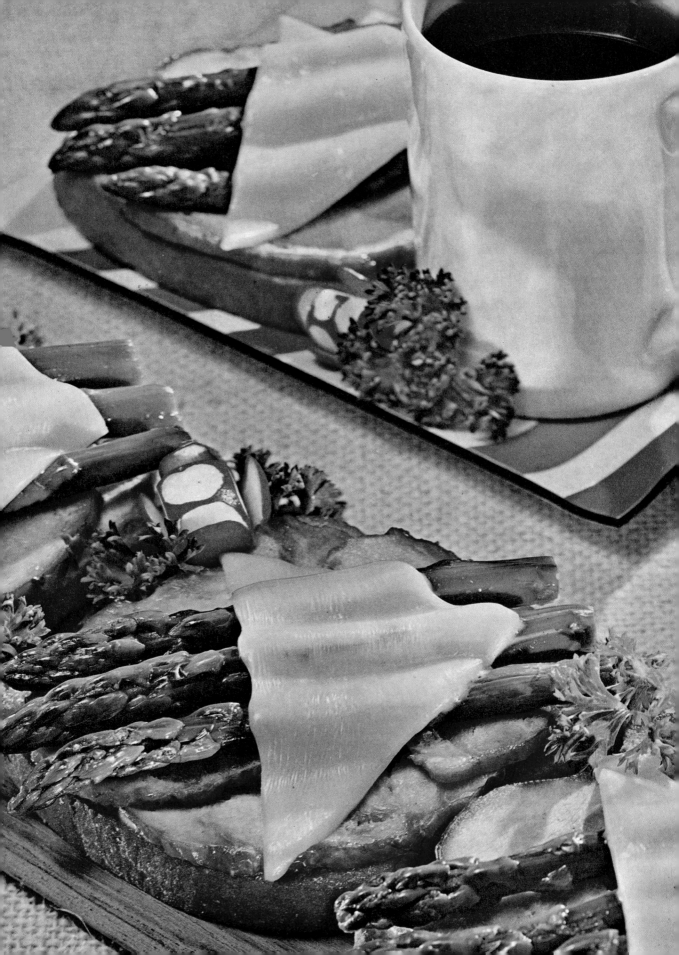

Luscious desserts

BAKED CUSTARD

■ ◣

    3 slightly beaten eggs
    ¼ teaspoon salt
    2 cups skim milk, scalded
    ½ to 1 teaspoon vanilla
       Non-caloric liquid sweetener equal
          to ¼ cup sugar

Combine eggs and salt. Slowly stir in slightly cooled milk, vanilla, and sweetener. Set six 6-ounce custard cups in shallow pan on oven rack. Pour hot water 1 inch deep around them. Pour in custard. Bake at 325° for 40 to 45 minutes or till knife inserted off-center comes out clean. Each serving equals ■ 1 Meat Exchange and ◣ ½ Milk Exchange. Top with fruit if desired.

COFFEE CHIFFON

◣

Soften 2 envelopes (2 tablespoons) unflavored gelatin in ½ cup cold water. In medium saucepan, beat 2½ cups skim milk and 3 egg yolks. Add non-caloric liquid sweetener equal to ½ cup sugar, 1 tablespoon instant coffee powder, ½ teaspoon salt, and softened gelatin.

Cook and stir till mixture thickens and gelatin is dissolved. Chill till partially set. Beat 3 egg whites, 1 teaspoon vanilla, and ¼ teaspoon cream of tartar till soft peaks form. Fold in gelatin mixture. Spoon into 6-cup mold. Chill firm. Makes 10 servings, each ◣ ½ Milk Exchange.

RICE RAISIN PUDDING

■ ◣

Combine 2 slightly beaten eggs, 2 cups cooked rice, 1 cup evaporated *skim* milk, non-caloric liquid sweetener equal to ½ cup sugar, ½ cup light raisins, ½ cup water, 1 teaspoon vanilla, ¼ teaspoon salt, and ¼ teaspoon ground cinnamon.

Set a 1½-quart baking dish in shallow pan on oven rack. Pour water 1 inch deep around dish. Pour pudding in baking dish. Bake at 350° for 45 minutes, or till knife inserted off-center comes out clean. Makes 8 servings each ■ 1 Bread Exchange and ◣ ½ Milk Exchange.

APPLE CRUNCH

■ ■ ■

Place 4 cups pared, sliced apples in a 1-quart casserole. Combine ¾ cup orange juice, non-caloric liquid sweetener equal to ½ cup sugar, 1 teaspoon ground cinnamon, and 1 teaspoon lemon juice. Pour over apples and toss.

Combine 1 cup graham-cracker crumbs with 2 tablespoons melted butter. Sprinkle over apples. Cover with foil and bake at 400° for 25 minutes. Uncover and bake 5 to 10 minutes longer. Serves 6, each ■ 1 Fruit Exchange, ■ 1 Bread Exchange, and ■ 1 Fat Exchange.

RIBBON FUDGE PARFAIT

■ ◣

    1 4-serving envelope low-calorie
          chocolate pudding mix
    2 teaspoons instant coffee powder
    1¾ cups skim milk
    2 stiffly beaten egg whites
    1 1¼-ounce envelope low-calorie
          dessert topping mix

In saucepan, combine pudding mix (dry) and instant coffee; slowly stir in milk. Cook and stir till mixture boils. Remove from heat; cool; beat smooth. Fold in stiffly beaten egg whites. Prepare topping mix according to package directions. Fold ½ *cup* topping into pudding. Alternately spoon pudding and remaining topping into 6 parfait glasses. Chill. Each parfait equals ■ 1 Fat Exchange and ◣ ½ Milk Exchange.

TAPIOCA PUDDING

◣

Combine 2 cups skim milk, 2 tablespoons quick-cooking tapioca, non-caloric liquid sweetener equal to 5 tablespoons sugar, and ¼ teaspoon salt. Let stand 5 minutes. Add 2 slightly beaten egg yolks. Bring to boil over medium heat, stirring constantly. Remove from heat (mixture will be thin); add ½ teaspoon vanilla.

Beat 2 egg whites to stiff peaks. Gradually fold in hot mixture. Chill. Serves 8. Each serving equals ◣ ½ Milk Exchange.

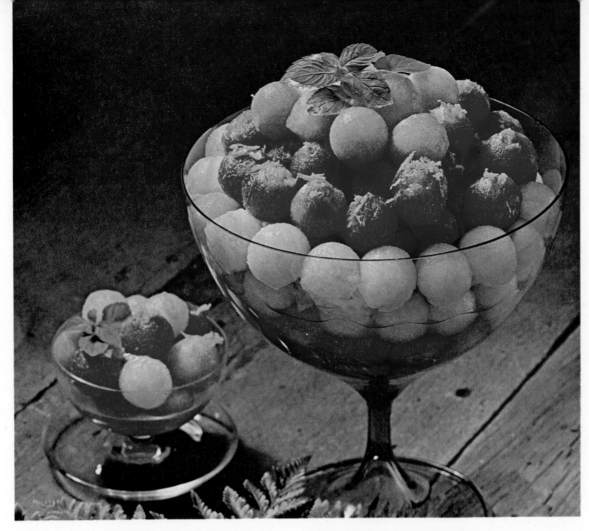

The delicate, sweet flavor of Rainbow Melon Julep is accented with a sparkling, tangy blend of juices and carbonated beverage. Garnish with a sprig of fresh mint.

RAINBOW MELON JULEP

2 teaspoons shredded orange peel
2 teaspoons shredded lime peel
½ cup orange juice
½ cup lime juice
  Non-caloric liquid sweetener equal to 2 to 4 tablespoons sugar
2 tablespoons chopped fresh mint
8 cups melon balls (watermelon, cantaloupe, honeydew)
1 cup low-calorie lemon-lime carbonated beverage, chilled

Combine peels, juices, sweetener, and mint; pour over melon balls; chill at least 2 hours. Just before serving, pour carbonated beverage over fruit. Garnish with mint sprigs. Makes eight 1-cup servings of ■ 1 Fruit Exchange each.

GREEN 'N GOLD COMPOTE

1 1-pound 4-ounce can dietetic-pack pineapple chunks
2 small fully ripe bananas
3 oranges
½ pound seedless green grapes
1 cup low-calorie lemon-lime carbonated beverage, chilled

Drain pineapple chunks, reserving liquid. Slice bananas on the bias into the liquid; drain. Pare and slice oranges, removing seeds. Halve slices. Wash grapes and divide in small clusters. Layer pineapple, bananas, and oranges. Mound grape clusters in center. Chill thoroughly. Just before serving, slowly pour chilled carbonated beverage over fruit. Makes 5 cups. Each ⅓-cup serving equals ■ 1 Fruit Exchange.

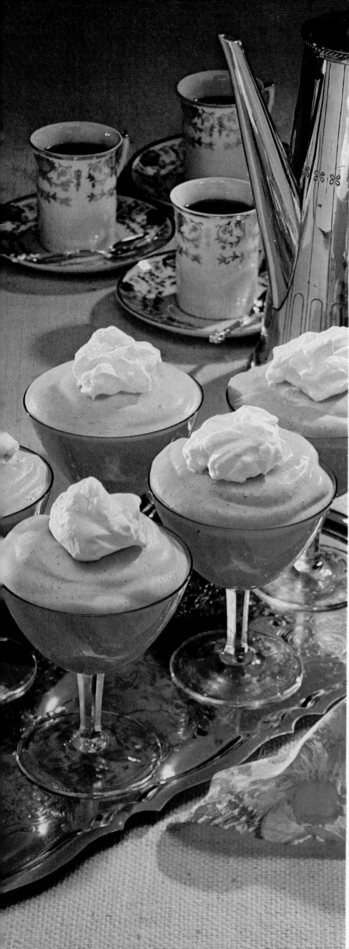

PLUM WHIP

- 1 envelope (1 tablespoon) unflavored gelatin
- ¼ cup cold water
- 1 1-pound can dietetic-pack red plums
- 6 to 8 drops red food coloring
- 1 tablespoon lemon juice
- 2 egg whites
- 1 1¼-ounce envelope low-calorie dessert topping mix

Soften gelatin in cold water. Sieve plums and juice into saucepan; heat till boiling. Add softened gelatin, food coloring, and lemon juice; stir till dissolved. Cool till partially thickened. Beat egg whites and dash salt till soft peaks form; add plum mixture gradually and beat till fluffy. Prepare topping according to package directions. Fold *half* into plum mixture. Use remaining topping as garnish. Serve at once. Makes 10 servings, each ■ 1 Fruit Exchange.

FROZEN ORANGE DESSERT

Freeze ½ cup evaporated *skim* milk in refrigerator tray until almost frozen at edges. Combine 1 slightly beaten egg yolk, non-caloric liquid sweetener equal to ¼ cup sugar, 2 tablespoons orange juice, ½ teaspoon grated orange peel, and dash salt.

In a cold mixing bowl, combine ice cold milk and 1 egg white. Using cold beaters, whip until soft peaks form; add 2 tablespoons lemon juice and beat to stiff peaks. Gradually add orange juice mixture at low speed. Pour into a 5½-cup ring mold. Freeze until firm. Unmold. Makes 6 servings, each ▲ ¼ Milk Exchange.

RHUBARB SAUCE

In saucepan combine 3 cups rhubarb, cut in 1-inch pieces, non-caloric liquid sweetener equal to ⅓ cup sugar, and ½ cup water. Cover and cook slowly till tender, about 5 minutes. Makes 6 servings, each a ■ Free Exchange.

As light as a soft breeze

← Pink, fluffy Plum Whip is perfect to serve for a luncheon, or to top off a hearty meal. Serve with dainty cups of demitasse.

PEACH PARFAIT

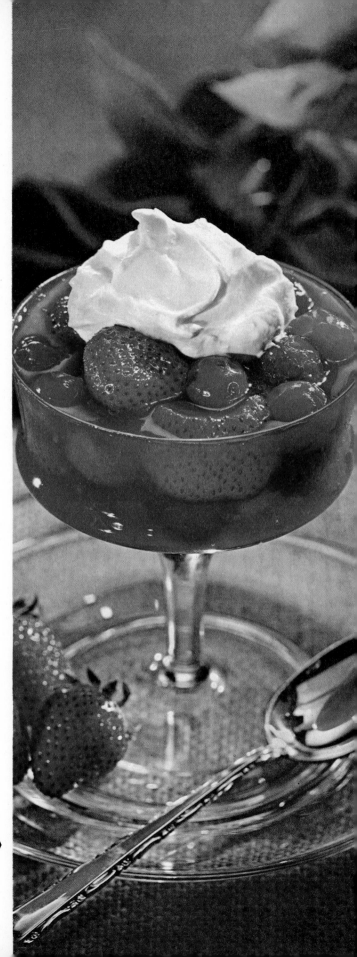

Prepare one 4-serving envelope raspberry-flavored low-calorie gelatin using package directions, but *use only 1½ cups water*. Mix one 1-pound can dietetic-pack peaches, drained and chopped, with *1 cup* gelatin; chill till partially set. Chill remaining gelatin till partially set.

Add ⅓ cup chilled evaporated *skim* milk and a few drops almond extract to gelatin *without* fruit. Whip till fluffy. Alternate the 2 gelatin mixtures in parfait glasses, ending with whipped gelatin. Serves 6, each ■ 1 Fruit Exchange.

FLUFFY WHIPPED TOPPING

Pour ⅓ cup evaporated *skim* milk into mixing bowl. Chill the bowl and beaters. Add non-caloric liquid sweetener equal to about 1 tablespoon sugar and ¼ teaspoon vanilla. Whip to stiff peaks. *Use immediately*. Makes 1¼ cups. Each ½ cup equals ▲ ¼ Milk Exchange.

RUBY FRUIT COMPOTE

1 1-pound can water pack pitted
   tart red cherries*
   Non-caloric liquid sweetener equal
     to ½ cup sugar
1 tablespoon cornstarch
   Dash salt
1 tablespoon lemon juice
4 drops red food coloring
   Dash bitters
1 pint fresh whole strawberries

Drain cherries, reserving liquid. Add water to cherry juice to make 1½ cups. Blend sweetener, cornstarch, salt, and cherry juice mixture. Cook stirring till thickened and bubbly. Add lemon juice, food coloring, bitters, and fruits. Chill. Serves 6. Each ⅔ cup serving is ■ 1 Fruit Exchange. If desired, top with 1 tablespoon sour cream equaling ▨ 1 Fat Exchange.

*To use fresh cherries, *substitute 1½ cups water* for cherry juice mixture.

A gem of a compote

**Ruby Fruit Compote is a sparkling, luscious →
blend of cherries and strawberries. Add a
dollop of sour cream for an extra treat.**

Beverages and snacks

HOT CHEESE AND CRAB DIP

■

Flake one 7½-ounce can crab meat. Cut in small pieces one 10-ounce stick sharp natural Cheddar cheese and one 8-ounce package sliced sharp process American cheese. Combine with ⅓ cup skim milk. Stir over low heat till cheeses melt. Add ½ cup sauterne and crab meat; heat through. Makes 3 cups. Two tablespoons dip equals ■ 1 Meat Exchange. Use vegetable dunkers or crackers from the Bread Exchange.

CREAMY COTTAGE DIP

■

Beat one 12-ounce carton (1½ cups) cottage cheese, not creamed, 6 tablespoons skim milk, 1½ teaspoons instant minced onion, and ½ teaspoon seasoned salt with electric mixer. Stir in 1 tablespoon finely chopped canned pimiento and 1 tablespoon snipped parsley. Chill. Makes 1¾ cups. Four tablespoons equals ■ 1 Meat Exchange. Good on baked potato too.

COCKTAIL WIENERS

■

1 pound frankfurters
1 12-ounce bottle extra hot catsup
2 teaspoons celery seed
1 tablespoon vinegar
1 clove garlic, halved

Diagonally slice each frankfurter in 6 pieces. Combine remaining ingredients and franks; cover and refrigerate for 4 hours. To serve, remove garlic; heat sauce and frankfurters. Six "wiener bites" equals ■ 1 Meat Exchange.

CHEDDAR SPREAD

■ ◣

Cube 8 ounces sharp natural Cheddar cheese at room temperature. Add ½ cup skim milk and 1 teaspoon prepared mustard. Beat with electric mixer until almost smooth. Serve with unpared apple wedges. Makes about 1 cup. Two tablespoons equal ■ 1 Meat Exchange; 5 apple wedges are ◣ ½ Fruit Exchange.

FROZEN BANANA MILK SHAKE

■ ◣

Peel 1 large firm ripe banana; slice into large chunks. Freeze. When frozen, combine in blender with 1 cup skim milk, non-caloric liquid sweetener equal to 2 tablespoons sugar, and dash nutmeg. Blend just till mixture is thick and frosty. Serve immediately. Makes 2 servings each ■ 1 Fruit and ◣ ½ Milk Exchange.

PEACHY LEMON SHAKE

■ ■ ◣

1 8-ounce can dietetic-pack peach slices
1 cup skim milk
⅔ cup lemon sherbet

Place peaches including juice in blender. Blend at high speed till smooth (about 10 seconds). Blend in milk. Add sherbet, mixing just till blended. Pour into 2 glasses. *Serve immediately.* Makes 2 servings each ■ 1 Fruit Exchange, ■ 1 Bread Exchange, and ◣ ½ Milk Exchange.

LIMEADE OR LEMONADE

■

5 cups water
1 cup lime juice *or* lemon juice
Non-caloric liquid sweetener equal to ½ to ¾ cup sugar

Combine all ingredients. Serve over ice. Garnish with mint sprigs and lime or lemon slices. Makes 6 cups. Each serving equals a ■ Free Exchange.

HOT COCOA

■

Mix 3 tablespoons cocoa (regular-type, dry), non-caloric sweetener equal to 3 tablespoons sugar, and ½ cup water. Bring to a boil, stirring constantly. Boil 1 minute. Add 3 cups skim milk; heat to boiling point (do not boil). Add ¼ teaspoon vanilla.

Beat with rotary beater just before serving. Makes 3 cups. Each ¾ cup serving equals ■ 1 Milk Exchange.

FRUITED ICED TEA

- 2 tablespoons instant tea powder
- 5 cups cold water
  Non-caloric liquid sweetener
  equal to ¼ cup sugar
- ½ cup orange juice
- ½ cup lime juice

Combine instant tea powder and the cold water; stir till tea is dissolved. Add sweetener, orange juice, and lime juice. Mix thoroughly. Chill. Serve over ice in tall glasses. Makes 6 servings, each a ■ Free Exchange. Garnish with orange slice and fresh cranberry.

SPICED PINEAPPLE SPARKLE

- 1½ cups water
- 6 inches stick cinnamon
- 12 whole cloves
  Non-caloric liquid sweetener equal
  to ½ cup sugar
- 1 46-ounce can pineapple juice
- 1½ cups orange juice
- ½ cup lemon juice
- 2 1-pint bottles low-calorie
  lemon-lime carbonated beverage

In saucepan, combine water, cinnamon, and cloves. Cover and simmer 15 minutes; strain. Cool. Add sweetener and fruit juices; chill. Just before serving, slowly pour in lemon-lime carbonated beverage. Serve over ice cubes with cinnamon stick muddlers. Makes 12 cups. Each ⅔ cup serving equals ■ 1 Fruit Exchange.

CRANBERRY COOLER

- 6 ice cubes
  Fresh strawberries, halved
- 1 quart low-calorie cranberry-
  juice cocktail, chilled
- 2 cups low-calorie lemon-lime
  carbonated beverage, chilled

Place ice cubes in a large pitcher. Add a few strawberries, then pour in cranberry-juice cocktail. Carefully pour low-calorie lemon-lime carbonated beverage down the side of the pitcher. Makes 6½ cups, each a ■ Free Exchange.

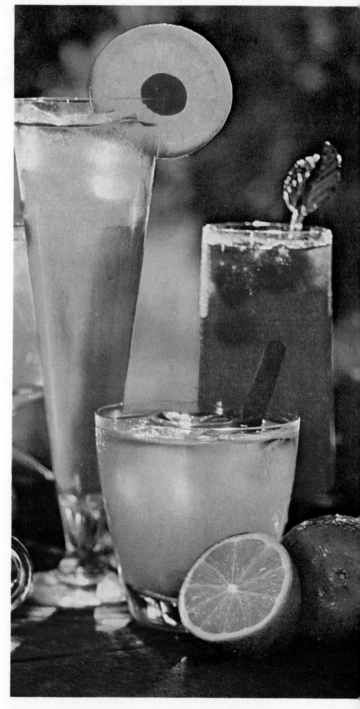

For a refreshing between-meal sipper, try Fruited Iced Tea served in a tall chilled glass or Cranberry Cooler with its pleasing strawberry floaters. Spiced Pineapple Sparkle, sporting a cinnamon stick stirrer, is a perfect punch for company.

CHAPTER 6

EATING OUT

Since the Food Exchange reducing diets in this book fit into normal patterns of living—no gimmicks, no exotic "wonder foods"—it's no trick at all to eat out without anyone's noticing that you're on a diet. In fact, it's better not to tell people you're dieting. It makes some hostesses uneasy.

Whether it's a private home dinner or restaurant dining, there are several ploys you can use to keep your calorie intake within bounds without being ostentatious about it.

You can leave fatty things on your plate—trimmed-off meat fat, thick gravies, rich toppings, breaded coatings, oils at the bottom of the salad bowl.

You can take large servings or seconds when green beans, spinach, broccoli, cauliflower, or asparagus are passed around. Heaps of these As Desired Vegetable Exchanges make it look as if you were a voracious eater.

As for cocktail hors d'oeuvres, nuts, little sausages wrapped in bacon, you can keep a little cache beside you and nobody will force refills on you.

There's a first-rate reducing menu in virtually every restaurant or cafeteria array of foods. And it's quite easy to find it when you apply the Food Exchange framework for reducing (page 27). Here is a representative restaurant menu, with reducer's choices indicated by an asterisk (*).

Eating in restaurants

If the chicken is fried with a delicious breaded crust, the crust can be peeled off with a knife and willpower and left untouched. Same goes for breaded fish and other similar foods.

Restaurants usually serve a basket of rolls and breads along with pats of butter. This will tempt you to nibble during the minutes before the main course arrives, so beware. Take *one* roll and *one* pat of butter (unless you'd rather save the butter for a baked potato), if allowed in your meal plan. Let the chilled butter soften on your plate so it will spread more thinly.

Sometimes, a cocktail precedes dinner at a restaurant, or elsewhere for that

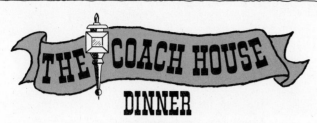

DINNER

APPETIZERS

Fresh Fruit Cup* Chilled Tomato Juice* French Onion Soup
Blue Point Oysters* Cherrystone Clams* Melon in Season*

CHEF'S SPECIALITIES

Chicken Ala Parisienne
A casserole, with fresh vegetables and mushrooms, under a
fluffy French pancake

Roast Stuffed Native Turkey*

Shish Kabob on Flaming Sword*
Wine-marinated beef tenderloin tips, broiled and served on
flaming skewer.

Roast Prime Rib of Beef Au Jus*
Roast Leg of Lamb with Mint Jelly*
Calf's Liver Saute with Bacon

SEAFOOD

Broiled Lobster Tail with Lemon Butter
Broiled Fresh Halibut*

STEAKS

Boneless New York Sirloin Steak*
Broiled Filet Mignon*
Chopped Sirloin of Beef with Onion Rings*

VEGETABLES

Asparagus* ◆ French-cut Green Beans* ◆ Garden Peas*
Whipped, Parsleyed, or Baked Potatoes*

SALADS

Fresh Fruit* ◆ Hearts of Lettuce* ◆ Molded Fruit Salad

Combination Salad Bowl*
Choice of French, Italian, Green Goddess or Vinegar and
Oil Dressing

DESSERTS

Home-made Apple Pie ◆ Pumpkin Pie ◆ Hot Mince Pie
Chocolate Brownie ◆ Plain Gelatin* ◆ Baked Apple*
Berries in Season* Watermelon* Ice Cream* and Sherbet*

BEVERAGES

Coffee* ◆ ◆ ◆ Tea* ◆ ◆ ◆ Milk*

Don't worry about that special dinner party. With the easy food exchange reducing plan, dining out is fun. Make your selections according to your daily meal plan using the 7 Menu Planning Steps.

Since ■ 1 Fruit Exchange is allowed for dinner, select an ■ As Desired Vegetable for an appetizer and a fruit for dessert.

Leave the dressing.

Trim off excess fat and order no gravy.
Leave the mint jelly.

For those with strong willpower, ¾ *cup* lobster may be eaten. Ask for hot seafood cocktail sauce for the lobster or halibut.

A steak usually weighs more than three ounces. Estimate your serving; and take the remainder home. Onion rings are taboo.

Request plain potatoes with a separate serving of butter. This controls the amount of butter added.

For dressing try vinegar, lemon or tomato juice.

One serving of plain gelatin equals ■ 1 Bread Exchange. Inquire if the baked apple is prepared without sugar. For ice cream count ■ 1 Bread Exchange and ■ ■ 2 Fat Exchanges.

*Reducer's choice.

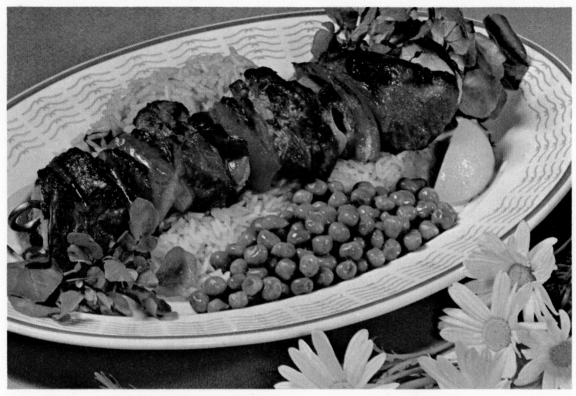

Enjoy eating out while continuing to lose weight. The chef's special Shish Kabob served on a skewer is a reducer's choice from The Coach House menu. A diner's menu is listed below.

matter. A low-calorie dinner can be converted into a fairly calorific one by "forgetting" to count alcoholic appetizers—discussed unflinchingly, page 38.

Dazzling wares of cafeterias, lined up for diners on the march, easily tempt to overloading a tray. There's a tendency to snatch in a hurry if people behind you are impatient. The thing to do is to window-shop first by sauntering outside the rail, noticing what's cooking and reading the itemized menu that is usually posted somewhere above the steam tables. With your mind made up, get into line, and pick just that.

The handy condensed Food Exchange Lists on the next page may be clipped out and carried in pocket or purse to aid you in eating out.

DINER'S CHOICE

- Tomato Juice
- Shish Kabob on Flaming Sword:
  - 3 ounces beef
  - tomato wedges
  - green pepper
  - ½ cup fluffy rice*
- ½ cup Garden Peas
- Combination Salad Bowl with Vinegar and Lemon
- Hard Roll† with 1 teaspoon Butter†
- 1 cup Strawberries with ½ cup Skim Milk
- Coffee

*On 1000 calorie diet omit the rice.
†Rolls and butter only fit into the 1500 calorie meal plan.

Food exchange lists

The Food Exchange Lists are eight groups of foods containing similar amounts of protein, fat, carbohydrate, and calories. The foods included are everyday favorites of the American diet. Each list has a color symbol for quick-as-a-glance recognition. The specified serving amount listed for each food item is equal to one food exchange.

Using a Daily Meal Plan on page 27, select foods you like from the respective Food Exchange Lists specified for each meal.

Your selections will automatically add up, in round numbers, to the number of calories in the meal plan you choose. Remember, you can substitute one food for another in the same food exchange list.

■ MEAT EXCHANGE ■

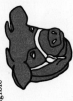

1 MEAT EXCHANGE EQUALS
Carbohydrate, negligible
Protein, 7 grams
Fat, 5 grams
Calories, 73

■ Cheese
American, Cheddar, Swiss: 1 ounce, 1 slice, 1 inch cube, ¼ cup grated
Cottage, not creamed, ¼ cup
■ Cold cuts, 1 slice
4½-inch diameter, ⅛-inch thick
Bologna
Braunschweiger
Luncheon loaf
Minced ham
Salami, Cotto
■ Eggs, 1
■ Fish
Cod, halibut, haddock, trout, snapper, etc., 1 ounce cooked
Crabmeat, lobster, ¼ cup
Sardines, 3 medium
Shrimp, clams, oysters, 5 small
Tuna, salmon, ¼ cup
■ Frankfurter, 1
■ Peanut butter, 2 tablespoons

■ Meat, poultry (no bone or visible fat)
1 ounce cooked or 3¼x2x¼-inch slice
Beef
Chicken
Corned beef
Ham
Lamb
Liver
Pork
Turkey
Veal

■ FREE EXCHANGE ■

1 FREE EXCHANGE EQUALS
Carbohydrate, negligible
Protein, negligible
Fat, negligible
Calories, negligible

May be used in any amount desired.

■ Bouillon
■ Broth, clear, fat free
■ Coffee
■ Cranberries
■ Gelatin, low-calorie
■ Gelatin, unflavored
■ Lemon
■ Mustard
■ Non-caloric sweetener, liquid, powder, or tablets
■ Pepper
■ Pickles, dill, unsweetened
■ Pickles, sour
■ Rennet tablets
■ Rhubarb
■ Spices
■ Tea
■ Vinegar

■ FRUIT EXCHANGE ■

1 FRUIT EXCHANGE EQUALS
Carbohydrate, 10 grams
Protein, negligible
Fat, negligible
Calories, 40

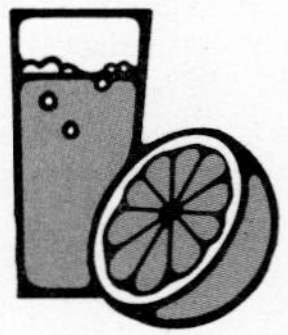

Raw, cooked, canned unsweetened, or frozen unsweetened
■ Apple, 1 (2-inch diameter)
■ Applesauce, ½ cup
■ Apricots*, dried, 4 halves
■ Apricots*, fresh, 2 medium
■ Banana, ½ small
■ Blackberries, 1 cup
■ Blueberries, ⅔ cup
■ Cantaloupe†*, ¼ (6-inch diameter)
■ Cherries, sour, ½ cup
■ Cherries, sweet, 10 large
■ Dates, 2
■ Figs, dried, 2
■ Figs, fresh, 2 large
■ Grape juice, ¼ cup
■ Grapefruit†, ½ small
■ Grapefruit juice†, ½ cup
■ Grapes, 12
■ Honeydew melon, ⅛ (7-inch diameter)
■ Mango†*, ½ small
■ Nectarine, 1 medium
■ Orange†, 1 small
■ Orange juice†, ½ cup
■ Papaya†, ¾ medium
■ Peach, 1 medium
■ Pear, 1 small
■ Pineapple, ½ cup cubed or 1 slice
■ Pineapple juice, ⅓ cup
■ Plums, 2 medium
■ Prunes, dried, 2 medium
■ Raisins, 2 tablespoons
■ Raspberries, 1 cup
■ Strawberries†, 1 cup
■ Tangerine, 1 large
■ Watermelon, 1 cup
†Rich sources of vitamin C.
*Rich sources of vitamin A.

■ FAT EXCHANGE ■

1 FAT EXCHANGE EQUALS
Carbohydrate, negligible
Protein, negligible
Fat, 5 grams
Calories, 45

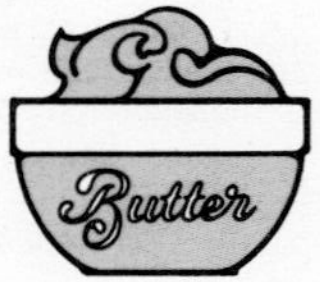

■ Avocado, ⅛ (4-inch diameter)
■ Bacon, crisp, 1 slice
■ Butter or margarine, 1 teaspoon
■ Diet-type margarine, 2 teaspoons
(For table use only, don't use in cooking.)
■ Cream, whipping (40%), 1 tablespoon
■ Cream, light (20%), 2 tablespoons
■ Cream cheese, 1 tablespoon
■ French or Italian salad dressing, 1 tablespoon
■ Mayonnaise, 1 teaspoon
■ Nuts, 6 small
■ Oils or shortening, 1 teaspoon
■ Olives, green, 5 small
■ Sour cream, 1 tablespoon

■ MILK EXCHANGE ■

1 MILK EXCHANGE EQUALS
Carbohydrate, 12 grams
Protein, 8 grams
Fat, negligible
Calories, 80

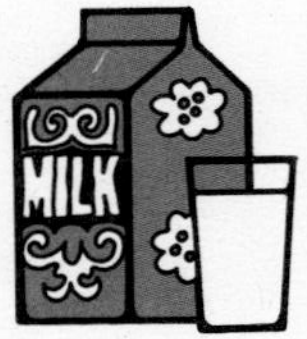

■ Buttermilk, from skim milk, 1 cup
■ Dried skim milk powder, ¼ cup
■ Dried whole milk powder‡, ¼ cup
■ Evaporated milk‡, ½ cup
■ Evaporated skim milk, ½ cup
■ Homogenized or whole milk‡, 1 cup
■ Plain yogurt‡, 1 cup
■ Skim milk, 1 cup
■ 2% butterfat milk**, 1 cup
‡Omit 2 Fat Exchanges from diet.
**Omit 1 Fat Exchange from diet.

SOUP

The following soups may be used in unlimited amounts as they are a ▮ Free Exchange:

Bouillon   Consomme   Clear broth

Other soups may be used in exchange for foods allowed in your diet. The following list shows the Exchanges for ½ *can of condensed soup* (before milk or water is added to the soup). Use milk in soups from the Milk Exchange.

Beef, ▮ 1 Bread Exchange and ▮ 1 Meat Exchange
Beef noodle, ▮ 1 Bread Exchange
Black bean, ▮ 2 Bread Exchanges
Chicken gumbo, ▮ 1 Bread Exchange
Chicken noodle, ▮ 1 Bread Exchange
Chicken rice, ▮ 1 Bread Exchange
Chicken vegetable, ▮ 1 Bread Exchange and ▮ 1 Fat Exchange
Clam chowder, Manhattan-style, ▮ 1 Bread Exchange and ▮ 1 Fat Exchange
Cream of asparagus, ▮ 1 Bread Exchange
Cream of celery, ▮ 1 Bread Exchange and ▮ 1 Fat Exchange
Cream of chicken, ▮ 1 Bread Exchange and ▮ 1 Fat Exchange
Cream of mushroom, ▮ 1 Bread Exchange and ▮ 2 Fat Exchanges
Cream of potato, ▮ 1 Bread Exchange
Green pea, ▮ 2½ Bread Exchanges
Minestrone, ▮ 1 Bread Exchange and ▮ 1 Fat Exchange
Onion soup, ▮ 1 Bread Exchange
Pepper pot, ▮ 1 Bread Exchange and ▮ 1 Meat Exchange
Scotch broth, ▮ 1 Bread Exchange and ▮ 1 Fat Exchange
Tomato, ▮ 1 Bread Exchange and ▮ 1 Fat Exchange
Turkey noodle, ▮ 1 Bread Exchange
Vegetable, ▮ 1 Bread Exchange
Vegetable beef, ▮ 1 Sturdy Vegetable Exchange and ▮ 1 Fat Exchange
Vegetarian vegetable, ▮ 1 Bread Exchange

Contributions to this list were made by the Greater Boston Diabetes Society, Inc.

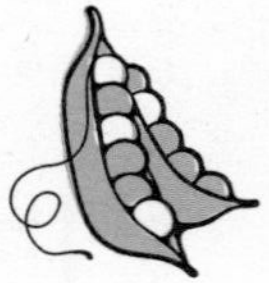

CRACKERS

Multi-shaped crackers, 11, ▮ 1 Bread Exchange and ▮ 1 Fat Exchange
Onion-flavored crackers, 10, ▮ 1 Bread Exchange and ▮ 1 Fat Exchange
Round cheese crackers, 6, ▮ 1 Bread Exchange and ▮ 1 Fat Exchange
Shredded wheat wafers, 3, ▮ 1 Bread Exchange
Small pencil-shaped Cheddar cheese crackers, 8, ▲ ½ Bread Exchange
Thin pretzel sticks, 30, ▲ ½ Bread Exchange
Thin triangle shaped crackers, 14, ▮ 1 Bread Exchange and ▮ 1 Fat Exchange
3-ring pretzels, 6, ▮ 1 Bread Exchange
Wheat wafers, 7, ▮ 1 Bread Exchange
For plain crackers see Bread Exchange List.

MISCELLANEOUS

Carbonated beverages, low-calorie, less than 5 calories per bottle, ▮ Free Exchange
Cranberry-juice cocktail, low-calorie, ½ cup, ▮ Free Exchange
Cranberry sauce, low-calorie, ½ cup, ▮ Free Exchange
Croutons, 1 cup, ▮ 1 Bread Exchange
Dessert topping mix, low-calorie, prepared according to package directions, ⅓ cup, ▮ 1 Fat Exchange
Fish sticks, frozen, 3 sticks, ▮ 1 Bread Exchange and ▮ 2 Meat Exchanges
Gelatin dessert, low-calorie, plain, ▮ Free Exchange
Mayonnaise, low-calorie, 2 tablespoons, ▮ 1 Fat Exchange
Pudding, low-calorie, made with skim milk according to package directions, ⅔ cup, ▮ 1 Milk Exchange
Salad dressings, less than 5 calories per tablespoon, commercial bottled, French, Italian, etc., ▮ Free Exchange
Soy sauce, ▮ Free Exchange
Tomato paste, 3 tablespoons, ▮ 1 Sturdy Vegetable Exchange
Tomato sauce, ¼ cup, ▮ 1 Sturdy Vegetable Exchange and ▮ 1 Fat Exchange
Vegetables, frozen in butter or cream sauce, ½ cup, ▮ or ▮ Appropriate Vegetable Exchange and ▮ 1 Fat Exchange

▮ BREAD EXCHANGE

▮ Bread, white, rye, whole wheat, 1 slice
Biscuit, 1 (2-inch diameter)
Cornbread, 1½-inch cube
English muffin, ½
Frankfurter bun, ½
Hamburger bun, ½
Melba toast, 7 rounds or 4 slices
Muffin, 1 (2-inch diameter)
Roll, 1 (2-inch diameter)
▮ Cake, plain and unfrosted angel or sponge, 1½-inch cube
▮ Cereal
Cooked, ½ cup
Dry, flaked or puffed, ¾ cup
▮ Crackers
Graham, 2 (2½-inch square)
Oysterettes, 20 (½ cup)
Round, thin, 6 to 8 (1½-inch diameter)
Rusks, 2
Saltines, 5 (2-inch square)
Soda, 3 (2½-inch square)
▮ Flour, 2½ tablespoons
▮ Ice Cream, ½ cup (omit 2 Fat Exchanges)
Noodles, spaghetti, cooked, ½ cup
Rice or grits, cooked, ½ cup

1 BREAD EXCHANGE EQUALS
Carbohydrate, 15 grams
Protein, 2 grams
Fat, negligible
Calories, 68

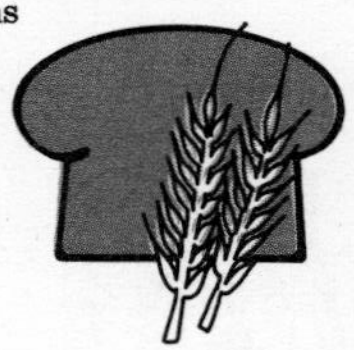

▮ Sherbet, ⅓ cup
▮ Vegetables
Baked beans, no pork, ¼ cup
Beans and peas, dried, cooked, ½ cup
black-eyed peas, kidney, lima, navy, split peas
Corn, popped (plain), 1 cup
Corn, sweet, ⅓ cup or ½ ear
Lima beans, fresh, cooked, ½ cup
Mixed vegetables, ½ cup
Parsnips, ⅔ cup
Potato, white, 1 (2-inch diameter) baked or boiled
Potato, white, mashed, ½ cup
Sweet potato or yam, ¼ cup

AS DESIRED VEGETABLE EXCHANGE ▮

Any amount may be eaten at each meal.

Asparagus
Bean sprouts
Beans, green or wax
Broccoli*†
Brussels sprouts
Cabbage
Cauliflower
Celery
Chickory*
Cucumber
Eggplant
Endive
Escarole*
Greens, all kinds* beet, chard, collard, kale, mustard, spinach
Lettuce
Mushrooms
Okra
Parsley
Pepper, green*†
Pimiento
Radish
Romaine
Sauerkraut
Squash, summer
Tomatoes*
Vegetable juice cocktail

*Rich sources of Vitamin A.
†Rich sources of Vitamin C.

1 AS DESIRED VEGETABLE EXCHANGE EQUALS
Carbohydrate, negligible
Protein, negligible
Fat, negligible
Calories, negligible

STURDY VEGETABLE EXCHANGE ▮

One serving equals ½ cup cooked vegetable or ½ cup raw vegetable.

Artichoke
Beets
Carrots*
Onions
Peas, green
Pumpkin*
Rutabaga
Squash, winter*
Butternut, acorn
Turnip

*Rich sources of Vitamin A.

1 STURDY VEGETABLE EXCHANGE EQUALS
Carbohydrate, 7 grams
Protein, 2 grams
Fat, negligible
Calories, 36

Lunches to carry

Lunch must sometimes be portable—stowed in a lunch box, desk drawer, or even an attaché case. A good sandwich *can* be about equal to the main course of a restaurant lunch—bread, vegetables, meat—combining several Food Exchanges in a well balanced mixed-diet package.

Mainstay sandwiches

Build a lunch-box meal around a hearty sandwich, such as:
• ■ Luncheon meat, ■ American cheese, thinly sliced ■ dill pickle, and ■ mustard on ■ hard roll.
• ■ Peanut butter and sliced ■ radish on ■ whole wheat bread.
• Thin slices of ■ tomato and ■ onion on ■ rye bread (wrap separately and assemble at lunchtime).
• Pared ■ cucumber slices and ■ low-calorie mayonnaise.
• ■ Meat or ham loaf with ■ catsup.
• Thin slices of ■ roast beef, ■ chicken, or ■ ham with ■ mustard, ■ catsup, or ■ low-calorie mayonnaise.
• ■ Hard-cooked egg with ■ pimiento, ■ celery, and ■ green pepper moistened with ■ low-calorie mayonnaise.
• ■ Tuna, ■ chopped celery, and ■ chopped apple moistened with a little ■ low-calorie mayonnaise.
• ■ Corned beef, ■ Swiss cheese, and thin slices of ■ dill pickle.

Sandwich Supplements

Round out the quality of a sandwich lunch with the following suggestions:
• Beverages: ■ milk, ■ tea, or ■ coffee (hot or iced), ■ lemonade, ■ fruit juice, ■ low-calorie carbonated beverages, ■ presweetened soft drink powders.
• Fruit: ■ apples, ■ oranges, ■ peaches, ■ plums, and ■ pears travel well. Pack ■ grapes in paper cups—no crushing. Or send chilled canned ■ fruits along in a wide-mouth vacuum jar. Remember to pack a plastic spoon for convenience, too.

• Relishes: ■ dill pickles, ■ radishes, thin ■ green pepper strips, ■ celery sticks, ■ carrot curls, and ■ cauliflowerets add crisp accent to the meal.
• Hot soup or ■ consomme can be carried in a vacuum bottle or purchased from a handy, nearby vending machine. (See Packaged Exchanges on page 31.)

Tips for lunch-box packers

• Fixing ■ roast beef or ■ ham sandwiches? Four or five paper-thin slices "bite" easier than one thick slice.
• Use a variety of ■ breads: white, rye, whole wheat, or French breads; English muffins or rolls; melba toast or crackers to go with soup.
• Spread ■ bread to the very edge with ■ butter or margarine to prevent a moist filling from soaking into the bread.
• Wrap ■ lettuce and ■ tomato slices separately in foil or clear plastic wrap so they will stay fresh, then put into the sandwich just before eating.
• Individual packages of ■ dill pickles from the store make packing easy.
• Score ■ orange and protect in clear plastic wrap—makes peeling a snap.
• Freeze a can of ■ tomato or ■ fruit juice for added variety. It will be thawed by lunchtime and, in the meantime, keeps the rest of the food cool.
• Pack ■ cottage cheese, ■ low-calorie pudding, or ■ low-calorie gelatin in wide-mouth vacuum jar. Plastic spoons come in handy for eating.
• Cut sandwiches in quarters—reducers will feel they are eating more.
• Save a serving for a snack— ■ fruit, ■ peanuts, a cool drink, or ■ crackers, and ■ cheese—later in the day.
• Make a week's supply of sandwiches at once (■ peanut butter, ■ chicken, and ■ meat freeze best). Wrap individually and pack all of one kind in a box; label with contents and date. Take wrapped sandwiches from freezer in the morning. They'll be just right for eating at lunch.

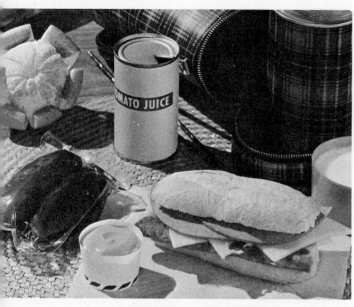

A crusty French roll filled with layers of meat, cheese, and lettuce makes a hearty meal-in-one sandwich for lunch-box eaters. Send mustard in small cup to spread on at lunchtime.

Tips for lunches-to-carry are useful at picnic time, too. Enjoy the festivities with grilled hamburgers served open-face on French bread. Pass crunchy celery, carrots, and radishes.

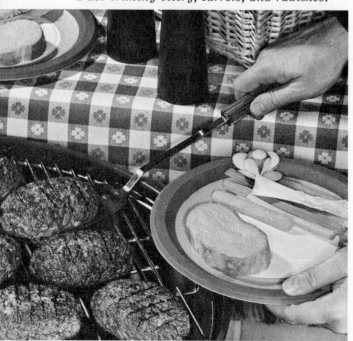

1500 CALORIE

MEAL PLAN

■ ■ ■ 3 Meat Exchanges
■ ■ 2 Bread Exchanges
■ As Desired Vegetable
■ 1 Fruit Exchange
■ 1 Milk Exchange
■ 2 Fat Exchanges
■ Free Exchanges

LUNCH BOX

■ Tomato Juice
Poor Boy Sandwich:
■ ■ 1 small brown-and-serve
French roll
■ 1 slice Bologna, halved
■ 1 slice boiled ham, halved
■ 1 slice Swiss cheese, halved
■ lettuce
■ 2 teaspoons butter
■ mustard
■ ■ 2 Dill Pickles
■ 1 small Orange
■ 1 cup Skim Milk

✳ EXCHANGE TIPS

In order to have 2 slices of bread for a sandwich at noon, 1200 calorie reducers may transfer 1 Bread Exchange from either breakfast or dinner to lunch. For variety, pack items separately and assemble an open-faced sandwich at lunch.

Reducers following the 1000 calorie meal plan may wish to save the 1 Bread Exchange at breakfast for an open-faced sandwich at lunch. Or try rolling slices of meat in lettuce leaves for a new twist.

Salad plates provide a nice change of pace. Pack cottage cheese and low-calorie gelatin in wide-mouth vacuum jar. Take along a selection of fresh fruit and lettuce packaged separately. Keep paper plates, plastic forks on hand at work.

CHAPTER 7

FAMILY STYLE REDUCING

If one member of the family needs to reduce and others do not, must two kinds of meals be prepared? No, not at all.

Cooking procedures scarcely need to be changed. Take a serving of vegetables from the pot for the reducer before adding cream or butter. Gravies, sauces, cream, sugar, butter, and salad dressings, are often served from separate containers at the table. Reducers can simply look the other way while non-reducers take all they want. Special low-calorie salad dressings can be purchased or prepared in advance (see recipes on page 56).

If family members crave home-fried potatoes, don't dream of depriving them. The reducer can take a piece of bread and get more or less the nutritional equivalent of the potatoes, minus the frying fats. In many other ways, a little knowledge about Food Exchanges enables easy substitutions to be made for favorite family foods that are too calorific for reducers.

Better Homes and Gardens Food Exchange reducing diets give a foundation of good daily nutrition for everybody.

All that's missing is calories. It's easy to build really good family meals around foods the reducer uses. Normal weight family members who need more calories just *add* wholesome foods the reducer must restrict: more bread, fats, whole milk products, sweets, pastries, cakes, cookies, and the like.

One menu expanded

The chart on the next page shows how easy it is. Additional foods for the family do not, of course, have to be exactly the ones listed.

Not very long from now—when you have slimmed down to normal weight—you'll need to add enough calories for a maintenance diet (see page 83). Then you can begin to add some of the same things that the chart allows as additions for family diet. Don't, however, add in amounts that make your weight rebound to the high side. What you learn by choosing foods from the family meals for reducing purposes will help a great deal to keep your weight permanently at its most flattering level.

A 1200 CALORIE DINNER
MENU FOR THE ENTIRE FAMILY

REDUCER'S MENU

■■■■ *Favorite Beef Loaf**
■ *1 Boiled New Potato with*
    1 teaspoon Butter

■ *Bean-stuffed Tomato**

CHERRY WHIP:

■ *10 large Cherries*
▲ *Fluffy Whipped Topping**

▲ *¼ cup Skim Milk*
■ *Coffee*

FAMILY MENU

Favorite Beef Loaf*
Boiled New Potatoes with
Cream Sauce
Glazed Carrots
Bean-stuffed Tomato*

CHERRY SHORTCAKE:

Sponge Cake
Cherries
Whipped Cream

Homogenized Milk
Coffee

*See recipe section

Don't spend all day in the kitchen just because someone in the family is reducing. Prepare one meal by making a few substitutions in the menu.

For example, prepare in the afternoon for the entire family Favorite Beef Loaf and Bean-stuffed Tomatoes. As the dinner hour approaches the only preparations left are the potatoes and carrots. Boil all the potatoes in one saucepan. Remove one serving of boiled potatoes before adding the cream sauce to the remaining potatoes, or pass the cream sauce in a small bowl.

Since one serving of Favorite Beef Loaf includes 1 Sturdy Vegetable Exchange, the carrots have been omitted from the reducer's menu.

End the meal with a luscious dessert served to all. Simply remove the shortcake and substitute Fluffy Whipped Topping for whipped cream.

Snacks and refreshments

Anything you "save" from your reducing diet, for in-between use when you feel the urge to eat, isn't really a snack. It's part of your diet, cleverly used to depress appetite by good timing.

But now and then you may want to add a snack that isn't on your diet-menu. This isn't immoral. It needn't even slow the speed of your reducing diet significantly if you choose a snack that is quite low in calories but temporarily gives a nice filled feeling. For example: a cup of bouillon or consomme; carrot and celery sticks; cauliflowerets, radishes, green pepper strips, and cabbage. Try sour or dill pickles; low-calorie carbonated beverages with less than five calories per bottle; plain low-calorie gelatin dessert; rhubarb sauce; tomato or vegetable juice cocktail.

CHAPTER 8

HOW TO STAY SLIM

Happy days are here when you have slimmed down to normal weight. That's the time to add some tasty calories to your meals. It isn't safe to keep on losing weight after you have no more excess fat to lose.

It's not immoral to be fat. It's uncomfortable and fatiguing and burdensome to body processes, but not immoral. So there's no reason in the world to feel constantly guilty about overweight or to look in a mirror and moan, "Who could love me?" and take a double banana split to ease unhappiness. There's every reason to *do* something about it, with absolute confidence that you will succeed if you establish a realistic calorie deficit.

After achieving normal weight, don't let 10 or 20 extra pounds pile on again and then go on a strict diet. By far the most successful way to stay slim for the rest of your life is to prevent small weight increases from becoming bigger ones. It's relatively easy. Decreasing caloric intake a mere 100 calories a day, or increasing exercise by that amount, can result in a loss of almost 10 surplus pounds a year. Take the long-term slim-silhouette point of view—and never be overweight again.

If you are proud of your new slim figure—*be proud!* You've earned it. It's a personal achievement, demonstrating willpower that skinny folk never have to exercise. The ego *should* inflate when weight deflates. See if it doesn't!

Keeping an inflated ego

Remember your fat is in your hands.

However, the battle of overweight isn't won once and for all by successful reducing. You want to stay that way. A tendency to gain weight usually lasts for a lifetime, and fat can come right back again if eating is wholly unrestrained. It is far better to stay slim than to go on repeated "reducing binges." Some people lose a hundred pounds or more a year, grasping at every new "wonder diet" that comes along, losing a few pounds and gaining it all back, over and over. Such crash reducing regimes are pretty stressful on body and psyche.

The treacherous thing about eating to maintain normal weight, after reducing, is that added foods may be unsuspectedly high in calories although they may not take up much stomach space. What you have learned about Food Exchanges in reducing will help you enormously to stay reduced. Foods provided are common to American diets. Through your own meal planning you have seen how they assure the essentials of good nutrition. This makes the transition to higher calorie diets easy and natural for you.

You can get the same balance of good nutrition but more calories by keeping the same *proportion* of Food Exchanges as in reducing. Simply increase the size of servings and add the use of sugar. The Maintenance Calorie Chart (page 17) can serve as a guide for the approximate calories needed to stay slim.

You can also add delicacies of your own choosing such as pie, cake, ice cream, other temptations. There is nothing disreputable about them. They're as good as the nutrients that go into them. Pies and cakes, for instance, contain such good things as cereals (flour), eggs, shortening, milk solids, fruit, plus a good deal of sugar. You'll recognize some of these components as members of the Bread, Fruit, Milk, Fat, and Meat Exchanges.

You have a few more calories to "spend" on a maintenance diet and can afford to indulge yourself within reason. A sure sign of over-indulgence is upward-creeping of the scales. Just keep tab on yourself and if weight seems to be getting out of hand again, use your knowledge of Food Exchanges to eat and stay slim the rest of your life.

You can be the master of your fat.

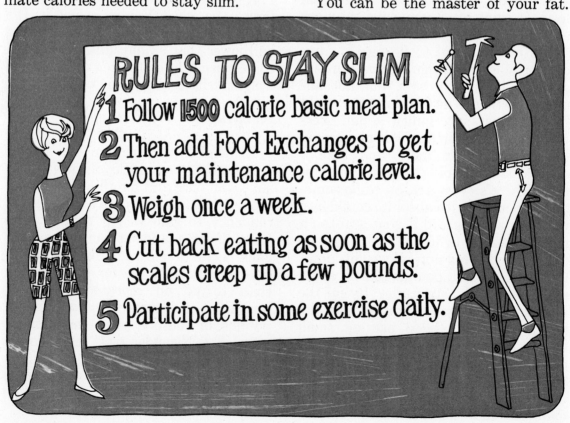

RULES TO STAY SLIM

1 Follow 1500 calorie basic meal plan.

2 Then add Food Exchanges to get your maintenance calorie level.

3 Weigh once a week.

4 Cut back eating as soon as the scales creep up a few pounds.

5 Participate in some exercise daily.

Daily exercises

Daily exercise for many people is greater during the warm seasons and dwindles as the temperature drops. To aid weight reduction, a non-seasonal program is recommended. The President's Council on Physical Fitness offers an exercise program perfect for every season of the year.

This physical fitness program is designed to firm flabby muscles. There should be no fear of developing large, unattractive bulges. Instead, your appearance will improve as muscles begin to provide better support. You'll feel full of vitality.

A daily routine of five workouts per week at the same time of day is ideal. Decide upon a time convenient for you—upon arising, in the middle of the day, or before retiring. Don't expect your physical fitness to change overnight. However, you will gradually feel more "alive," energetic, and at ease in doing the daily exercises.

A slight feeling of soreness the morning after the workout is one sign that flabby muscles have been exercised. To avoid this pain the program has levels of exercises. The Step 1 Exercises work all muscles gradually. When these exercises are done without fatigue and "rest stops," you are ready to advance to Step 2 Exercises.

Types of exercises

There are three types of exercises at each level: the warm-up, the conditioning, and the circulatory. The warm-up exercises stretch and limber the muscles. They prepare the body for greater exertion and decrease unnecessary strain which causes soreness. The same six exercises are used as warm-up exercises at both levels.

The conditioning exercises firm flabby abdominal, back, leg, and arm muscles. When you've mastered these exercises, you're ready to progress to Step 2.

One special exercise each workout serves to strengthen circulation and respiration. These circulatory activities contract large muscle groups and therefore can be done for longer periods of time than the other exercises.

The object of this exercise program is to proceed as fast as you can within your own limitations. Your age, health, and previous conditioning will determine your ultimate goal. Since you are competing with yourself, you can proceed at your own pace. Remember there's no race against time.

The daily workout

A chart included at each exercise level lists the number of repetitions for each exercise. If you can't do all the repetitions, stop and rest, then continue the count. Start slowly so that progress won't be interrupted by soreness. After completing the warm-up exercises, proceed to the conditioning exercises. End each workout with one circulatory activity of your choice.

From workout to workout fewer rest periods will be needed, and therefore the time spent for each workout will be shorter. As your speed increases be careful to perform each exercise correctly—don't rush through the workout. To add variety and fun to the daily workout, do the exercises to music or with family members. Caution: remember you are competing against yourself, not against a family member.

How do you know when to leave Step 1 Exercises and proceed to Step 2? The second level of conditioning has been reached when all the exercises can be done without fatigue and interruptions for rest. This advance can occur after a minimum of one week or five workouts. If you feel any strain while doing the beginning exercises, don't hesitate to spend two or three weeks on the first level.

Once the feeling of vitality has been achieved, maintaining this energy is easy. Just keep the previous routine of five workouts per week or a minimum of three exercise workouts per week.

If your daily exercises are discontinued for more than a week due to illness, begin at a lower level of repetition. Start slowly and gradually build up—in a short period of time the original level of physical fitness will again be reached.

Women: step 1 exercises

WARM-UP EXERCISES AND REPETITIONS

1. Bend and Stretch......................10
2. Knee Lift...............10 left, 10 right
3. Wing Stretcher........................20
4. Half Knee Bend.....................10
5. Arm Circles................15 each way
6. Body Bender...........10 left, 10 right

CONDITIONING EXERCISES AND REPETITIONS

7. Prone Arch...........................10
8. Knee Push-up.........................6
9. Head and Shoulder Curl...............5
10. Ankle Stretch......................15

CIRCULATORY ACTIVITIES (choose one each workout)

Walking...½ mile
Rope (skip 15 seconds, rest 60 seconds)...................................3 series

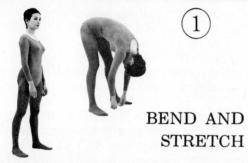

① BEND AND STRETCH

Do this exercise slowly; stretch and relax at intervals rather than in rhythm.
Starting Position: Stand erect with feet shoulder-width apart.
Count 1. Bend trunk forward and down, flexing knees. Stretch gently in attempt to touch fingers to toes or floor.
Count 2. Return to starting position.

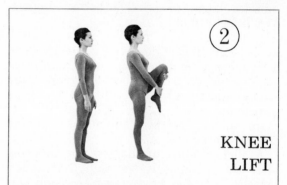

② KNEE LIFT

Starting Position: Stand erect with feet together and arms at sides.
Count 1. Raise left knee as high as possible; grasp leg with hands and pull knee against body while keeping back straight.
Count 2. Lower to starting position.
Counts 3 and 4. Repeat with right knee.

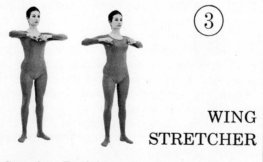

③ WING STRETCHER

Starting Position: Stand erect, elbows at shoulder height, fists clenched at chest.
Count 1. Thrust elbows backward vigorously without arching back. Keep head erect, elbows at shoulder height.
Count 2. Return to starting position.

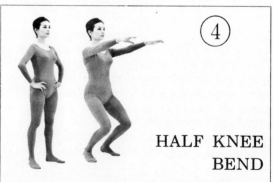

④ HALF KNEE BEND

Starting Position: Stand erect with feet shoulder-width apart and hands on hips.
Count 1. Bend knees halfway while extending arms forward with palms down.
Count 2. Return to starting position.

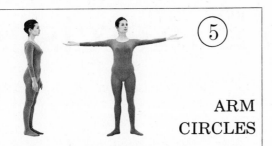

ARM CIRCLES

Starting Position: Stand erect, arms extended sideward at shoulder height, palms up.
Count 1. Make 15 small circles backward with hands. Keep head erect.
Count 2. Reverse, turn palms down and do 15 small circles forward.

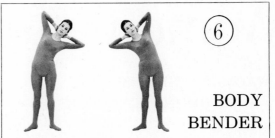

BODY BENDER

Starting Position: Stand, feet shoulder-width apart, fingers interlaced behind neck.
Count 1. Bend trunk sideward to left as far as possible, keeping hands behind neck.
Count 2. Return to starting position.
Counts 3 and 4. Repeat to the right.

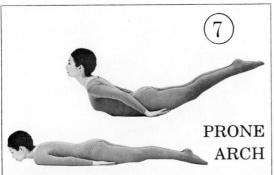

PRONE ARCH

Starting Position: Lie face down with hands tucked under thighs.
Count 1. Raise head, shoulders, and legs from floor.
Count 2. Return to starting position.

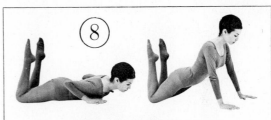

KNEE PUSH-UP

Starting Position: Lie face down with legs together. Bend knees raising feet off floor. Place hands, palms down, under shoulders.
Count 1. Push upper body off floor until arms are fully extended and body is in straight line from head to knees.
Count 2. Return to starting position.

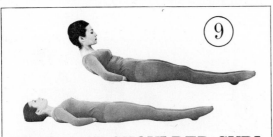

HEAD AND SHOULDER CURL

Starting Position: Lie on back, hands palms down and tucked under small of back.
Count 1. Tighten abdominal muscles, lift head pulling shoulders and elbows off floor. Hold for four seconds.
Count 2. Return to starting position.

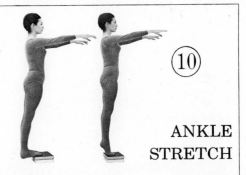

ANKLE STRETCH

Starting Position: Stand on a stair, large book, or block of wood, heels raised, with weight on balls of feet.
Count 1. Lower heels.
Count 2. Raise heels.

WALKING: Step off at a lively pace, swing arms, and breathe deeply. ROPE: Any form of skipping or jumping is acceptable. Gradually increase the tempo as your skill and condition improve.

Women: step 2 exercises

WARM-UP EXERCISES (first 6 exercises from step 1 exercises)

CONDITIONING EXERCISES REPETITIONS
1. Toe Touch...5
2. Sprinter..8
3. Sitting Stretch..10
4. Knee Push-up...8
5. Sit-up (arms extended)..5
6. Leg Raiser...5 each leg
7. Flutter Kick...20
8. **CIRCULATORY ACTIVITIES** (choose one each workout)
Walking (120 steps a minute)...................................½ mile
Rope (skip 30 seconds; rest 60 seconds)......................2 series
Run in Place (run 50, straddle hop 10) 2 cycles.............2 minutes

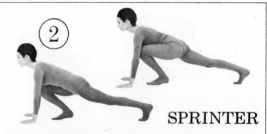

① TOE TOUCH

Starting Position: Stand at attention.
Count 1. Bend trunk forward and down; keep knees straight; touch fingers to ankles.
Count 2. Bounce and touch fingers to feet.
Count 3. Bounce and touch fingers to toes.
Count 4. Return to starting position.

② SPRINTER

Starting Position: Squat, placing hands on floor with fingers pointed forward. Extend left leg fully to rear.
Count 1. Reverse position of feet in bouncing movement. Bring left foot to hands, extend right leg backward—all in one motion.
Count 2. Reverse feet again, returning to starting position.

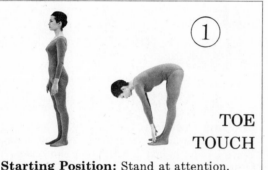

③ SITTING STRETCH

Starting Position: Sit with legs spread apart, hands on knees.
Count 1. Bend forward at waist, extending arms as far forward as possible.
Count 2. Return to starting position.

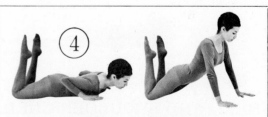

④ KNEE PUSH-UP

Starting Position: Lie face down with legs together. Bend knees raising feet off floor. Place hands, palms down, under shoulders.
Count 1. Push upper body off floor until arms are fully extended and body is in straight line from head to knees.
Count 2. Return to starting position.

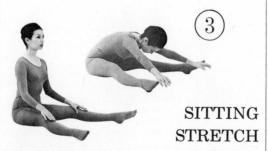

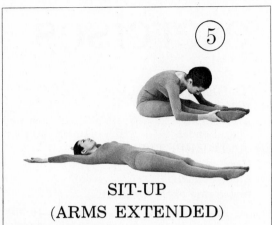

SIT-UP
(ARMS EXTENDED)

Starting Position: Lie on back, legs straight and together, arms extended beyond head.
Count 1. Bring arms forward over head, roll up to sitting position, sliding hands along legs, grasping ankles.
Count 2. Roll back to starting position.

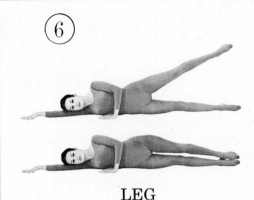

LEG
RAISER

Starting Position: Lie with right side of body on floor, head resting on right arm.
Count 1. Lift left leg 24 inches off floor.
Count 2. Lower left leg to starting position. Repeat 5 times. Repeat on left side.

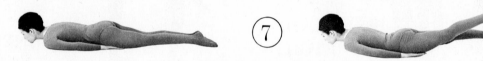

FLUTTER KICK

Starting Position: Lie face down with hands tucked under thighs.
Count 1. Arch the back, raising chest and head. Kick from hips with knees slightly bent, moving legs 8 to 10 inches apart. Flutter kick continuously; each kick counts as one.

At each workout choose one of the following:
WALKING: Set a pace of 120 steps per minute for ½ mile. Swing arms; breathe deeply.
ROPE: Skip or jump rope continuously using any form for 30 seconds, then rest 60 seconds. Repeat 2 times.
RUN IN PLACE: Raise each foot at least 4 inches off the floor and jog in place. Count 1 each time left foot touches floor. Complete number of running steps called for in chart, then do specified number of straddle hops. Complete 2 cycles of alternate running and straddle hopping for time specified on chart.
STRADDLE HOP
Starting Position: Stand at attention.
Count 1. Swing arms sideward and upward, touching hands above head (arms straight) while simultaneously moving feet sideward and apart in a single jumping motion.
Count 2. Spring back to starting position. Two counts in one hop.

CIRCULATORY
ACTIVITIES

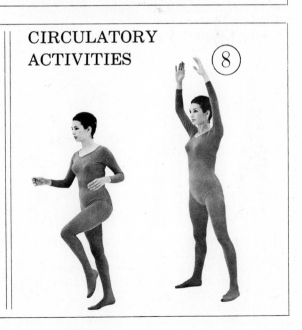

Men: step 1 exercises

WARM-UP EXERCISES AND REPETITIONS

1. Bend and Stretch....................10
2. Knee Lift...............10 left, 10 right
3. Wing Stretcher........................20
4. Half Knee Bend....................10
5. Arm Circles................15 each way
6. Body Bender............10 left, 10 right

CONDITIONING EXERCISES AND REPETITIONS

7. Prone Arch..........................10
8. Knee Push-up........................6
9. Head and Shoulder Curl...............5
10. Ankle Stretch.....................15

CIRCULATORY ACTIVITIES (choose one each workout)

Walking...½ mile
Rope (skip 15 seconds, rest 60 seconds)...3 series

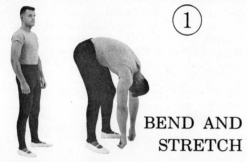

① BEND AND STRETCH

Do this exercise slowly; stretch and relax at intervals rather than in rhythm.
Starting Position: Stand erect with feet shoulder-width apart.
Count 1. Bend trunk forward and down, flexing knees. Stretch gently in attempt to touch fingers to toes or floor.
Count 2. Return to starting position.

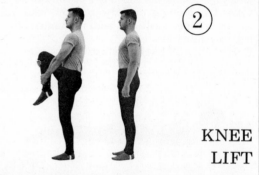

② KNEE LIFT

Starting Position: Stand erect with feet together and arms at sides.
Count 1. Raise left knee as high as possible; grasp leg with hands and pull knee against body while keeping back straight.
Count 2. Lower to starting position.
Counts 3 and 4. Repeat with right knee.

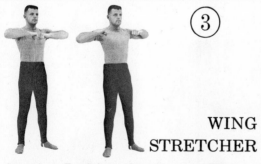

③ WING STRETCHER

Starting Position: Stand erect, elbows at shoulder height, fists clenched at chest.
Count 1. Thrust elbows backward vigorously without arching back. Keep head erect, elbows at shoulder height.
Count 2. Return to starting position.

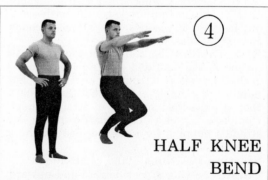

④ HALF KNEE BEND

Starting Position: Stand erect with feet shoulder-width apart and hands on hips.
Count 1. Bend knees halfway while extending arms forward with palms down.
Count 2. Return to starting position.

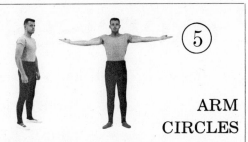

ARM CIRCLES

Starting Position: Stand erect, arms extended sideward at shoulder height, palms up.
Count 1. Make 15 small circles backward with hands. Keep head erect.
Count 2. Reverse, turn palms down and do 15 small circles forward.

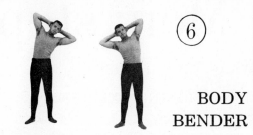

BODY BENDER

Starting Position: Stand, feet shoulder-width apart, fingers interlaced behind neck.
Count 1. Bend trunk sideward to left as far as possible, keeping hands behind neck.
Count 2. Return to starting position.
Counts 3 and 4. Repeat to the right.

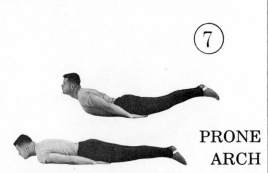

PRONE ARCH

Starting Position: Lie face down with hands tucked under thighs.
Count 1. Raise head, shoulders, and legs from floor.
Count 2. Return to starting position.

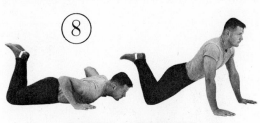

KNEE PUSH-UP

Starting Position: Lie face down with legs together. Bend knees raising feet off floor. Place hands, palms down, under shoulders.
Count 1. Push upper body off floor until arms are fully extended and body is in straight line from head to knees.
Count 2. Return to starting position.

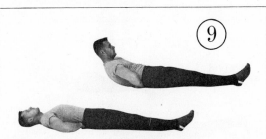

HEAD AND SHOULDER CURL

Starting Position: Lie on back, hands palms down and tucked under small of back.
Count 1. Tighten abdominal muscles, lift head pulling shoulders and elbows off floor. Hold for four seconds.
Count 2. Return to starting position.

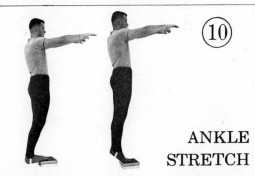

ANKLE STRETCH

Starting Position: Stand on a stair, large book, or block of wood, heels raised, with weight on balls of feet.
Count 1. Lower heels.
Count 2. Raise heels.

WALKING: Step off at a lively pace, swing arms, and breathe deeply. ROPE: Any form of skipping or jumping is acceptable. Gradually increase the tempo as your skill and condition improve.

Men: step 2 exercises

WARM-UP EXERCISES

(first 6 exercises from step 1 exercises)

CONDITIONING EXERCISES   **REPETITIONS**

1. Toe Touch...10
2. Sprinter...12
3. Sitting Stretch..12
4. Push-up..4
5. Sit-up (arms extended)...5
6. Leg Raiser..12 each leg
7. Flutter Kick...30
8. CIRCULATORY ACTIVITIES (choose one each workout)
Walking (120 steps a minute)..1 mile
Rope (skip 30 seconds, rest 30 seconds)..........................2 series
Run in Place (run 60, straddle hop 10) 2 cycles...........2 minutes

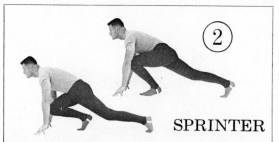

① TOE TOUCH

Starting Position: Stand at attention.
Count 1. Bend trunk forward and down; keep knees straight; touch fingers to ankles.
Count 2. Bounce and touch fingers to feet.
Count 3. Bounce and touch fingers to toes.
Count 4. Return to starting position.

② SPRINTER

Starting Position: Squat placing hands on floor with fingers pointed forward. Extend left leg fully to rear.
Count 1. Reverse position of feet in bouncing movement. Bring left foot to hands, extend right leg backward—all in one motion.
Count 2. Reverse feet again, returning to starting position.

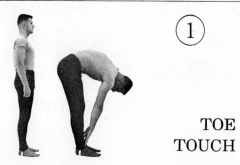

③ SITTING STRETCH

Starting Position: Sit with legs spread apart and hands on knees.
Count 1. Bend forward at waist, extending arms as far forward as possible.
Count 2. Return to starting position.

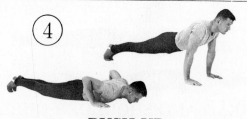

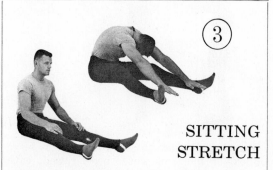

④ PUSH-UP

Starting Position: Lie on floor, face down, legs together, hands on floor under shoulders with fingers pointing straight ahead.
Count 1. Push body off floor by extending arms, so that weight rests on hands and toes.
Count 2. Lower the body until chest touches floor. Note—body should be kept straight.

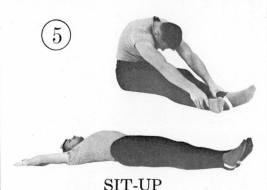

SIT-UP
(ARMS EXTENDED)

Starting Position: Lie on back, legs straight and together, arms extended beyond head.
Count 1. Bring arms forward over head, roll up to sitting position, sliding hands along legs, grasping ankles.
Count 2. Roll back to starting position.

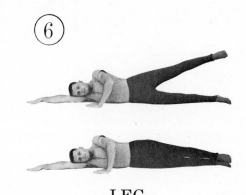

LEG
RAISER

Starting Position: Lie with right side of body on floor, head resting on right arm.
Count 1. Lift left leg 24 inches off floor.
Count 2. Lower left leg to starting position. Repeat 12 times. Repeat on left side.

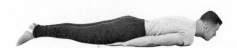 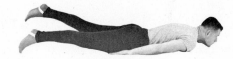

FLUTTER KICK

Starting Position: Lie face down on floor with hands tucked under thighs.
Count 1. Arch the back, raising chest and head. Kick from hips with knees slightly bent, moving legs 8 to 10 inches apart. Flutter kick continuously; each kick counts as one.

At each workout choose one of the following:
WALKING: Set a pace of 120 steps per minute for 1 mile. Swing arms; breathe deeply.
ROPE: Skip or jump rope continuously using any form for 30 seconds, then rest 30 seconds. Repeat 2 times.
RUN IN PLACE: Raise each foot at least 4 inches off the floor and jog in place. Count 1 each time left foot touches floor. Complete number of running steps called for in chart, then do specified number of straddle hops. Complete 2 cycles of alternate running and straddle hopping for time specified on chart.
STRADDLE HOP
Starting Position: Stand at attention.
Count 1. Swing arms sideward and upward, touching hands above head (arms straight) while simultaneously moving feet sideward and apart in a single jumping motion.
Count 2. Spring back to starting position. Two counts in one hop.

CIRCULATORY
ACTIVITIES

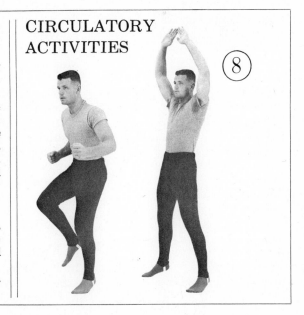

INDEX

A—C

Alcohol slows
progress, 38
Appetizers, 52-53
Apple Crunch, 68
-applesauce Mold,
Lime, 54
Artichokes, Marinated, 52
As Desired Vegetable
Exchange, 24, 30, 34
Banana Milk Shake,
Frozen, 72
Barbecue, Ham, 60
Barbecued Pork And
Beans, 60
Bean-stuffed
Tomatoes, 57
Beef Fillets,
Pampered, 61
Beef Loaf, Favorite, 60
Beef-o-mato Soup, 53
Beef Patties, Deviled, 65
Beverages, 52-53, 72-73
Beverages,
alcoholic, 38
Body builds, 10-12
Bread Exchange, 24, 30, 33
Bread Stuffing, 58
Broiled Tomatoes, 57
Cabbage Pineapple
Slaw, 54
Calorie deficit,
daily, 16
Carbohydrate, 21
Cheddar Spread, 72
Cheese And Crab Dip,
Hot, 72
Chef's Salad, 64
Chicken Breasts,
Curried, 58
Chicken, French
Herbed, 58
Chili Con Carne, 64
Cocktail, Double Deck, 52
Cocktail Sauce,
Seafood, 53
Cocktail Wieners, 72
Cocoa, Hot, 72

Coffee Chiffon, 68
Compote, Green 'n Gold, 69
Compote, Ruby Fruit, 71
Corned-beef Dinner, 60
Corned Beef Slawich, 66
Cottage Cheese
Dressing, 54
Cottage Dip, Creamy, 72
Cranberry Cooler, 73
Cranberry Waldorfs,
Molded, 54
Cucumber-dill Sauce, 62
Cucumber Salad,
Blender, 54
Cuke-buttermilk Soup, 53
Curried Chicken
Breasts, 58
Custard, Baked, 68

D—H

Daily calorie deficit, 16
Daily Meal Plans, 27
Desserts
Apple Crunch, 68
Coffee Chiffon, 68
Compote, Green 'n
Gold, 69
Custard, Baked, 68
Fruit Compote, Ruby, 71
Fudge Parfait,
Ribbon, 68
Melon Julep, Rainbow, 69
Orange Dessert,
Frozen, 70
Peach Parfait, 71
Plum Whip, 70
Rhubarb Sauce, 70
Rice Raisin Pudding, 68
Tapioca Pudding, 68
Topping, Fluffy
Whipped, 71
Deviled Beef Patties, 65
Deviled Swiss Steak, 61
Diet
1500 calorie, 27, 48-51
1000 calorie, 27, 40-43
1200 calorie, 27, 44-47
Dip, Creamy Cottage, 72

Dip, Hot Cheese And
Crab, 72
Dressing
Cottage Cheese, 54
Gourmet, 56
Slim-trim, 56
Tomato, 56
Exchange, Food,
explanation, 23-26, 32-37
Exchange Lists, Food, 28-31
Exchange Lists, Food,
clip-out, 77-78
Exercise, general, 17-19
Exercises, daily, 85-93
Fad diets, 8, 14
Family menus, 81-82
Fat Exchange, 29, 36
Fats, 21
1500 calorie
diet, 27, 48-51
Flounder In Wine, 62
Fluid retention, 22
Food Exchange, ex-
planation, 23-26, 32-37
Food Exchange Lists, 28-31
Frank-vegetable
Medley, 64
Free Exchange, 28, 37
French Herbed Chicken, 58
Fruit Compote, Ruby, 71
Fruit Exchange, 24, 29, 35
Fruited Iced Tea, 73
Fudge Parfait, Ribbon, 68
Gazpacho, 53
Gourmet Dressing, 56
Ham Barbecue, 60

I—M

Iceberg Ring, 55
Jamaican Swizzle, 52
Lamb Chops Oriental, 62
Limeade or Lemonade, 72
Lime-applesauce Mold, 54
Loaf, Favorite Beef, 60
Lunches to carry, 79-80
Macaroni And Cheese, 64
Main Dish Seasoning
Guide, 58

Main dishes, 58-67
Maintenance Calorie
    Chart, 17
Maintenance
    calories, 16-17
Maintenance
    diet, 26, 83-84
Marinated Artichokes, 52
Meal Plans, Daily, 27
Meat Exchange, 24, 25, 28,
    32
Melon Julep, Rainbow, 69
Menu
    family, 82
    1500
        calorie, 49-51, 76, 80
    lunch-box, 80
    1000 calorie, 41-43, 76
    planning, 39
    restaurant, 75, 76
    1200
        calorie, 45-47, 76, 82
Milk
    Exchange, 24, 25, 29, 36
Mixed dishes, 25-26, 52-73
Molded Cranberry
    Waldorfs, 54
Mushrooms, Pickled, 52

N—R

Nutrition, elements of
    good, 20
1000 calorie
    diet, 27, 40-43
Orange Dessert,
    Frozen, 70
Overweight, signs of, 9
Packaged Exchanges, 31
Pampered Beef
    Fillets, 61
Peach Parfait, 71
Peachy Ham Swisser, 66
Peachy Lemon Shake, 72
Perfection Salad, 54
Pickled Mushrooms, 52
Pills, reducing, 15
Pineapple Passion, 53
Pineapple Sparkle,
    Spiced, 73
Pizza, No Crust, 65
Plateau, losing, 21
Plum Whip, 70
Poached Salmon, 62

Pork And Beans,
    Barbecued, 60
Pot Roasts,
    Individual, 60
Potato Salad, Potluck, 57
Protein, 20
Pudding, Rice
    Raisin, 68
Pudding, Tapioca, 68
Rarebit, Welsh, 64
Reducing speed,
    approximate, 17
Restaurant dining, 74-76
Rhubarb Sauce, 70
Rice Raisin Pudding, 68

S

Salad
    Bean-stuffed
        Tomatoes, 57
    Cabbage Pineapple
        Slaw, 54
    Chef's, 64
    Cucumber, Blender, 54
    Iceberg Ring, 55
    Lime-applesauce Mold, 54
    Molded Cranberry
        Waldorfs, 54
    Perfection, 54
    Potato, Potluck, 57
    Tuna, 55
    Tuna, Slim-jim, 64
Salad Supper Sandwich, 66
Salmon Bake, Smoked, 62
Salmon, Poached, 62
Sandwiches
    Beef Patties,
        Deviled, 65
    Corned Beef Slawich, 66
    Peachy Ham Swisser, 66
    Salad Supper
        Sandwich, 66
    Skilletburgers, 65
    Tuna Salad Sandwich, 66
    Turkey-cheese
        Sandwich, 66
Sauce
    Cucumber-dill, 62
    Seafood Cocktail, 53
    Tartare, 62
Seafood Cocktail Sauce, 53
Seasoning Guide, Main
    Dish, 58

Seasoning Guide,
    Vegetable, 56
Shake, Frozen Banana
    Milk, 72
Shake, Peachy Lemon, 72
Skillet Spaghetti, 60
Skilletburgers, 65
Slaw, Cabbage
    Pineapple, 54
Smoked Salmon Bake, 62
Snacks, 72-73, 82
Soup, Beef-o-mato, 53
Soup, Cuke-buttermilk, 53
Spaghetti, Skillet, 60
Spiced Pineapple
    Sparkle, 73
Stuffing, Bread, 58
Sturdy Vegetable
    Exchange, 24, 30, 34
Swiss Steak, Deviled, 61
Swizzle, Jamaican, 52

T—W

Tapioca Pudding, 68
Tartare Sauce, 62
Tea, Fruited Iced, 73
Tomato Dressing, 56
Tomato Refresher, 52
Tomatoes, Broiled, 57
Topping, Fluffy
    Whipped, 71
Tuna Salad, 55
Tuna Salad
    Sandwich, 66
Tuna Salad, Slim-jim, 64
Turkey-cheese
    Sandwich, 66
1200 calorie
    diet, 27, 44-47
Vegetable
    Exchanges, 24, 30, 34
Vegetable Seasoning
    Guide, 56
Water and
    overweight, 15
Water retention, 22
Weight chart, men, 12
Weight chart, women, 11
Weight loss, time of
    greatest, 21
Weight record, weekly, 96
Welsh Rarebit, 64
Wieners, Cocktail, 72

4-16-79

SCORE YOUR PROGRESS

Record your weekly goal under the "desired" heading. Score your weight on the same day of the week under the "actual" heading opposite your weight goal for that week.

Desired	Actual	Desired	Actual	Desired	Actual	Desired	Actual
	193						